AF800799

ORTHOPAEDIA: SPINE

Produced by:

THE CODMAN GROUP

Orthopaedia is produced by The Codman Group (a 503C IRS-approved public charity) in collaboration with the United States Bone and Joint Initiative and the Community of Musculoskeletal Educators. ***Orthopaedia*** aims to serve as a free, up-to-date, peer-reviewed open educational resource for students and practitioners, thereby improving the welfare of patients.

Please visit *http://www.orthopaedia.com* for the most current version of this text. At the website, you will also find its sister publications covering Sports Medicine, Hand, and Foot & Ankle disorders, Pediatrics, and others as they become available.

Dan Jacob, *President, The Codman Group*

Joseph Bernstein, MD, FACS
Stephen J. Pinney, MD, MEd, FRCS(C)
Christian Veillette, MD, FRCS(C)
Orthopaedia Editors

Orthopaedia: Spine by CODMAN Group is licensed under a Creative Commons Attribution-NonCommercial-ShareAlike 4.0 International License, except where otherwise noted.

CONTENTS

PREFACE

Back pain is the most common symptom prompting people to seek medical care. In the United States alone, there are more than 50 million patient visits annually for spine related complaints. Moreover, approximately 1% of the American workforce is disabled because of chronic back or neck problems. One study examining spending on personal health care and public health in the United States (JAMA. 2016;316(24):2627-2646) estimated that the cost of caring for back pain exceeds the spending on care for asthma, breast cancer, cirrhosis, heart failure and leukemia – combined.

Back pain often originates from degenerative changes, but in many instances the precise cause is unknown. Intervertebral disc degeneration and facet joint arthritis is frequently seen in people without symptoms too.

Back pain is not the only spinal condition of interest either. The spine can also be affected by acute trauma, infection, tumor, and deformity.

It's important that I disclose my potential biases. I am an orthopaedic surgeon, working in a neurosurgical unit. I have seen that decompressive spinal surgery can be extremely gratifying for patients, producing near-immediate relief of arm pain or leg pain. After spine surgery done well, patients can experience complete resolution of pre-operative pain, sending a smile across their faces, even when groggy in the post-anesthesia recovery room. Operative fixation of spinal fractures can also have similar awe-inspiring results.

Of course, I have also seen that done poorly, spinal surgery can produce less-rewarding results. I refer not only to infrequent but understandable complications such as infection, dural tears, or nerve root injury, but also to the harmful impact of indiscriminate and unnecessary procedures. The rate of spinal fusion surgery has surged over the last 2 decades, a change driven at least in part by the medical industrial spinal complex.

Accordingly, this volume is not a treatise on spine surgery, but rather an introduction to spinal disorders, aiming to present a sound anatomical and physiological basis for understanding these important conditions.

There is no doubt that our understanding is incomplete, and hopefully subsequent editions will fill in the gaps. In the meanwhile, I am pleased to help share what we do know.

–Nader M. Hebela, MD

A WORD ON PEER REVIEW

There is a great profusion of medical information available for free on the Internet, and a lot of it is good. Yet even good information may not be completely useful to the reader who may not know if it is trustworthy. By contrast, there is also a lot of medical information available for sale that is produced by well-known authors and organizations, though not always for free.

This volume aims to be both free and accurate.

To ensure medical accuracy, each chapter was reviewed by an attending orthopaedic surgeon expert who was not involved in the creation of the material. These reviewers were asked to read the chapter with one overriding goal in mind: to detect errors. We are grateful to the following reviewers, all of whom offer their assurance that the chapter under their review is a fair, reasonable and valid representation of the topic for medical students, devoid of gross errors of omission or commission.

PEER REVIEWERS

- Adolescent Idiopathic Scoliosis was reviewed by Michael Glotzbecker, MD
- Ankylosing Spondylitis and Other Spondyloarthropathies was reviewed by Andrew Milby, MD
- Burners and Stingers was reviewed by Andrew Milby, MD
- Cervical Radiculopathy and Myelopathy was reviewed by Malcolm Ecker, MD
- Early Onset Scoliosis was reviewed by Lindsay Andras, MD
- Lumbar Disc Disease was reviewed by Jonathan Grauer, MD
- Lumbar Spondylosis was reviewed by Peter Derman, MD
- Scheuermann's kyphosis was reviewed by Jeff Sawyer, MD
- Spinal Infection was reviewed by Elizabeth Ames, MD
- Spinal Trauma & Spinal Cord Injury: General Principles was reviewed by Eric O Klineberg, MD
- Spinal Trauma & Spinal Cord Injury: Specific Injuries was reviewed by Malcolm Ecker, MD
- Spondylolysis and Spondylolisthesis was reviewed by Andrew Milby, MD

Further, to help ensure clarity (and help copy-edit as well) each chapter was reviewed by a medical student who was not involved in the creation of the material. We are grateful to the following Medical Student Reviewers: Jacob Ghahremani, Nathan Hasbani, Omair Kazi, Oscar Shen, Dennis Sievers, and Emily Wilson.

A NECESSARY DISCLAIMER

Peer-review notwithstanding, this being 21st century America, we must include the following Disclaimer, similar to those found in works produced by well-known authors and organizations.

This material was prepared for educational purposes only. We therefore disclaim any and all liability for any damages resulting to any individual which may arise out of the use of the material presented here. We similarly disclaim responsibility for any errors or omissions or for results obtained from the use of information contained here.

This material is not intended to represent the only, nor necessarily best, method or procedure appropriate for the medical situations discussed, but rather is intended to present an approach which may be helpful to others who face similar situations. We cannot can take any responsibility for the consequences following the application of any of the information presented here.

The information provided here cannot substitute for the advice of a medical professional. *Even if a given statement is completely true in the abstract, it may not apply to a given patient.*

The information we offer is provided "as is" and without warranty of any kind.

LIST OF CONTRIBUTORS

Orthopaedia: Spine was produced by editing, refining and merging material from many individual contributions and from other chapters within Orthopaedia. The specific and substantial contribution of three contributing editors listed below is acknowledged. They generously contributed first drafts and even more generously allowed their work to be edited, refined and merged (according to the overall needs of the project).

Steve Sungwon Cho, MD, MS
Barrow Neurological Institute

Scott M. LaValva, MD
Hospital for Special Surgery

Sara Weintraub, MD
Hospital of the University of Pennsylvania

EDITORIAL ASSISTANCE

We are grateful for the expert editorial help provided by Megan Flinner, www.ManagedByMegan.com

COVER ART

Cover art designed and donated by:

Louis C. Okafor, MD

louisokafor@gmail.com

CHAPTER 1.

ADOLESCENT IDIOPATHIC SCOLIOSIS

Scoliosis is a rotational deformity of the spine in both the coronal and sagittal planes (Figure 1). A diagnosis of idiopathic scoliosis is made when the coronal plane Cobb angle (see Figure 2) is >10 degrees on plain film radiographs and there is no underlying spinal cord pathology, neuromuscular disorder, or congenital malformation present. Adolescent idiopathic scoliosis is diagnosed in children between the ages of 10 and 18 years old and represents 80 percent or more of all cases. (Historically, if scoliosis is diagnosed in a patient 4 years of age or younger, it would be designated 'infantile idiopathic scoliosis' with the term 'juvenile idiopathic scoliosis' referring to patients ages 4-10, but more recently all cases of scoliosis diagnosed before the age of 10 are classified as 'early onset scoliosis' [discussed in another chapter.])

Depending on the severity of the curve and age of the patient, scoliosis can be managed with observation, bracing, or surgery. While scoliosis is not generally associated with pain during adolescence, more advanced curves (>40 degrees) can be associated with higher rates of low back pain in adulthood.

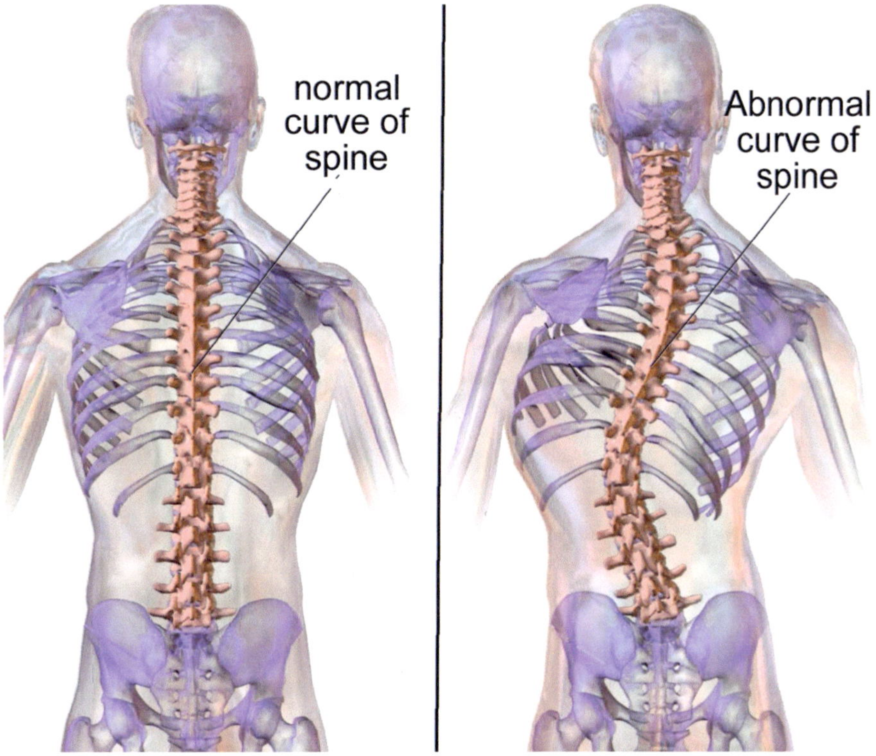

Figure 1: A normal spine and one with scoliosis (Images from Medical gallery of Blausen Medical 2014. WikiJournal of Medicine 1 (2). DOI:10.15347/wjm/2014.010. ISSN 2002-4436. https://commons.wikimedia.org/w/index.php?curid=27796937)

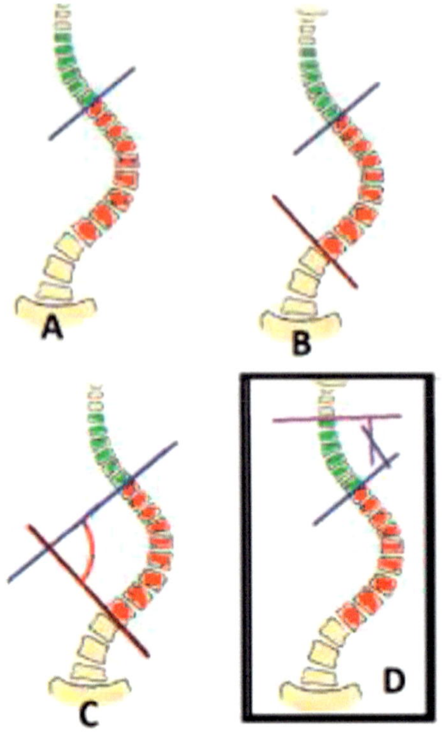

Figure 2: The magnitude of a scoliosis curve is given by the Cobb angle. To measure the Cobb angle, one must first identify the "end vertebrae," the top and bottom-most vertebral bodies in the curve. (As shown in the figure, this spine has 2 offsetting curves, denoted by green and red vertebral bodies.) Lines are then drawn along the superior endplate of the highest vertebral body (A) and the inferior endplate of the lowest vertebral body (B). These lines are then extended until they intersect; the angle between them is the Cobb angle (C). For smaller curves, the angle may be sufficiently small that the lines may not intersect on the films. In that case, the lines are extended only a short distance, but perpendicular lines are drawn from each towards the other line (as shown in D). The intersection of these perpendiculars (owing to geometry's rule of similar triangles) likewise defines the Cobb angle. The curves shown here are approximately 40 and 90 degrees. (Modified from Wikipedia).

STRUCTURE AND FUNCTION

The spine consists of 7 cervical, 12 thoracic, 5 lumbar, and 5-7 sacro-coccygeal vertebrae. Normal alignment is critical to maintain the balance of the axial skeleton between the head and pelvis. This alignment is measured in both the coronal and sagittal plane using a plumb line starting at the base of C7. In neutral coronal balance, the C7 plumb line overlaps the center of the sacrum. When the C7 plumb line is to the left of the sacrum, there is negative coronal balance and when it is to the right there is positive coronal balance. In neutral sagittal balance the C7 plumb line touches the posterior-superior corner of S1. If the C7 plumb line falls anterior to S1 there is positive sagittal balance, and if it falls posterior to S1 there is negative sagittal balance.

In the coronal plane, the spine should be straight (<10 degrees of curvature), but on the sagittal plane the lumbar spine typically has 20-55 degrees of lordosis (inward curving, as seen from the side), while the thoracic spine has a physiologic kyphosis (an outward curve or hunching of the spine) of 20-45 degrees.

PATIENT PRESENTATION

Adolescent idiopathic scoliosis is classically described as a painless condition. Low back pain is becoming increasingly more common among adolescent patients, and some of them will have scoliosis; but scoliosis should not be the default explanation of the symptoms.

A common complaint of adolescent idiopathic scoliosis patients is the appearance of the back and posture from a pronounced rib "hump," trunk shift, and uneven shoulders. Appearance issues can range from mild dysphoria to debilitating psychosocial distress.

Scoliosis may progress with growth. It is therefore important to establish the patient's growth history and document growth at each follow-up visit. On average, boys grow until the age of 16 and girls grow until the age of 14, or 2 years after menarche. Predicting growth is difficult, but some tools to help predict remaining growth include the Risser sign and Sanders stage (discussed below).

A complete physical exam begins with inspection of the patient standing upright facing away from the examiner. Scapular prominence, waist crease asymmetry and arm-side space can be observed. From a lateral view, the hypokyphosis of the thoracic spine can also be noted. Shoulder asymmetry, trunk shift and pelvic asymmetry can be observed and palpated. During the examination, it is important to identify a potential leg length discrepancy that can mimic scoliosis. If leg length difference is noted, the examiner can place a block under the shorter leg to assess if the curve corrects.

The Adam's forward bending test is an easy screening test. It is performed by having the patient lock his or her knees in extension and attempt to bend forward and touch toes. The patient is then observed from behind, to note the presence of an asymmetries of the rib cage and shoulder blades. Any rib prominence should be measured using a scoliometer (Figure 3). A rib prominence deformity greater than 7 degrees should prompt an evaluation by a pediatric spine specialist. As a rule of thumb, 7 degrees of prominence on Adam's forward bending test corresponds curve measuring about 10 to 20 degrees on x-ray.

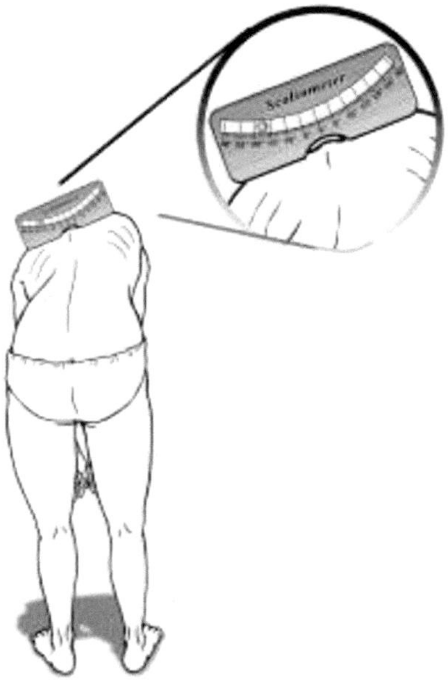

Figure 3: The Adams forward bending test. (A scoliometer, as shown, is nothing more than a carpenter's level with a cutout to rest on the spine and markings to indicate the angular deviation from the horizontal.) (Modified under a Creative Commons Attribution 4.0 International License from Application of two-parameter scoliometer values for predicting scoliotic Cobb angle. BioMed Eng OnLine 16, 136 (2017). https://doi.org/10.1186/s12938-017-0427-7)

OBJECTIVE EVIDENCE

There are important radiographic parameters to help with diagnosis and management of adolescent idiopathic scoliosis:

- Cobb angle: The angle between intersecting lines drawn perpendicular to the two end vertebrae (see Figure 1).
- End Vertebrae: Top and bottom vertebrae maximally tilted into the concavity.
- Neutral vertebra: Vertebra that are not rotated. Identified by symmetric pedicles in the coronal radiograph.
- Stable vertebra: Most cephalad vertebra distal to end vertebra that is most closely bisected by the central sacral vertical line.
- Apical vertebrae: Central vertebra within a curve, typically least tilted and most rotated.
- Risser sign: Radiographic predictor of growth based on the amount of iliac crest apophysis ossification (Figure 4).
- Sanders staging: Radiographic predictor of growth based on hand x-ray (Figure 5). In general, the bone epiphysis in the hand fuse from distal (phalangeal bones) to proximal (distal radius) and thus supports a staging system that ranges from 1 (skeletally immature) to 8 (skeletally mature).

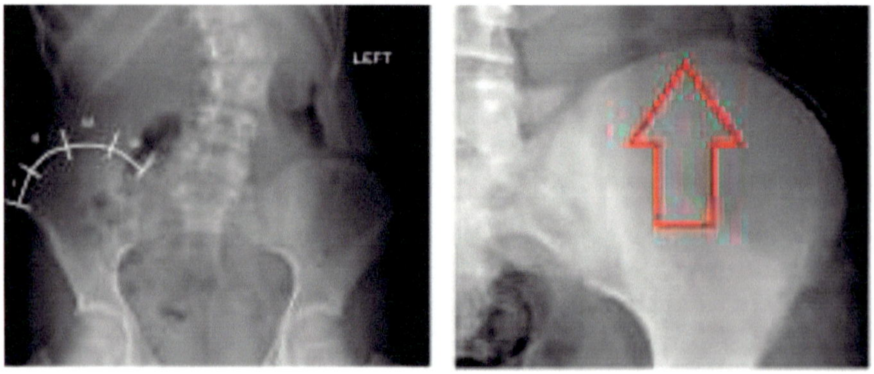

Figure 4: The Risser classification grades skeletal maturity based on the degree of ossification of the iliac crest apophyses. It begins with Risser Stage 0, where there is no ossification center at the level of iliac crest apophysis, and ends with stage 5, where there is complete ossification. Stages 1, 2, 3 and 4 are defined as 0 to 25% ossification, 25 to 50% ossification, 50 to 75% ossification, and 75% but less than 100% ossification, respectively. A Risser Stage 0 is shown in the x-ray at left, with a line indicating where the Stages 1 to 4 are defined. At right, a pelvic x-ray shows a Risser Stage 3 apophysis (Case courtesy of Dr Bruno Di Muzio, Radiopaedia.org, rID: 38297)

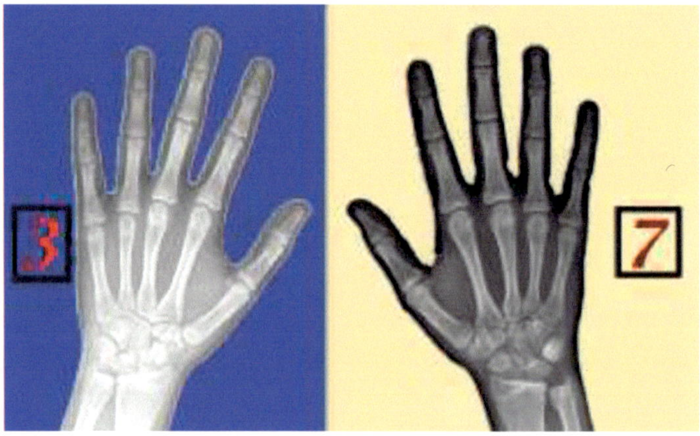

Figure 5: A hand x-ray corresponding to Sanders Stage 3 on the left and Stage 7 on the right. Note that in Stage 7, all physes are closed except for the distal radius physis, whereas the phalangeal and metacarpal physes are open in Stage 3.

EPIDEMIOLOGY

Adolescent idiopathic scoliosis is relatively rare, with a prevalence of 3% in the general population. The prevalence of severe curves (>30) is much lower, approximately 0.03%. When considering only large curves, females are ten times more commonly affected than males, but the ratio is closer to 1:1 for cases with smaller curves.

There is thought to be a genetic component to adolescent idiopathic scoliosis, though the mode of inheritance is unknown. The risk of having adolescent idiopathic scoliosis is increased 50-fold when both parents have a history of scoliosis. In females whose mother has a curve >15°, the risk is 27%.

DIFFERENTIAL DIAGNOSIS

So-called neuromuscular scoliosis is found when there are irregular spinal curvatures in the presence of the central nervous system or muscular disorders. In contrast to adolescent idiopathic scoliosis, neuromuscular curves tend to progress more rapidly, involve more vertebral levels, progress after maturity, and are usually associated with pelvic obliquity.

Scheuermann's Kyphosis is a spinal deformity causing rigid thoracic hyperkyphosis (>45 degrees). In general, adolescent idiopathic scoliosis is associated with "flat back," or loss of normal kyphosis and lordosis.

A leg length discrepancy can cause an apparent scoliosis. If present, leg length discrepancy will result in pelvic obliquity, and with it, a compensatory curve to keep the head and upper body over the center of the pelvis (see Figure 6).

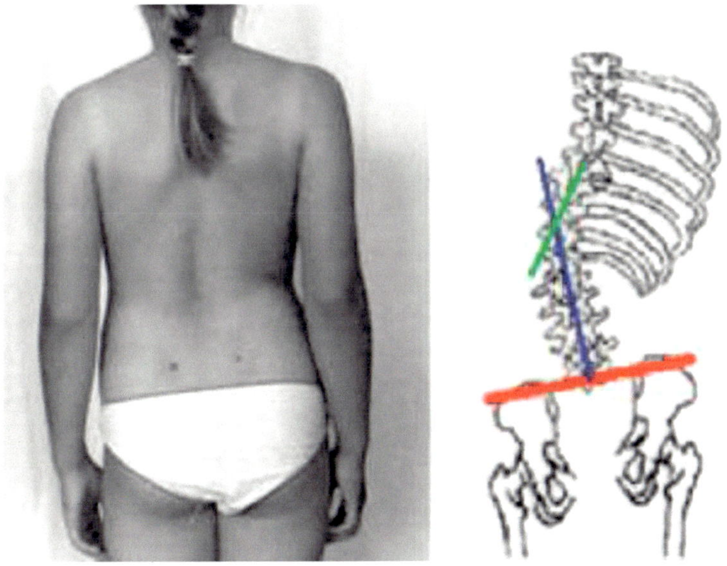

Figure 6: At left, a photograph of a patient with pelvic obliquity. This is defined (in the diagram at right) by the red line drawn across the iliac crests. The lumbar spine is accordingly tilted as well (blue line), with a compensatory curve above (intersection of green and blue lines) to keep the head centered over the body. (modified from https://www.ncbi.nlm.nih.gov/pmc/articles/PMC3282518/)

RED FLAGS

It is important to identify red flags during adolescent idiopathic scoliosis evaluation, which will warrant further investigation such as MRI to assess for intraspinal abnormalities such as syrinx, Chiari malformation, or cord tethering that may need to be addressed prior to curve correction. These include left thoracic curves (right thoracic curves are far more common), apical kyphosis (kyphosis is rare in adolescent idiopathic scoliosis), rapid progression of a curve, structural abnormalities such as a hemivertebrae, neurologic findings such as pathologic reflexes or radicular pain, and foot deformities.

TREATMENT OPTIONS AND OUTCOMES

The plan of treatment depends on the severity of the curve and patient age. After achieving skeletal maturity, curves <30 degrees are unlikely to progress in adulthood. In contrast curves >50 degrees are likely to progress 1 degree per year; and even higher rates are seen during pregnancy and menopause.

Curves smaller than 20 degrees have a low probability of progressing and require only surveillance with periodic physical exams until skeletal maturity. (After skeletal maturity is reached, curves smaller than 20 degrees do not need close monitoring.)

Curves measuring more than 20 degrees on initial presentation require intervention. The goal in treating patients with curves of more than 20 degrees but less than ~50 degrees (see Figure 7) is to prevent progression – not correction. This goal can often be achieved with thoraco-lumbar bracing. A landmark multicenter, prospective, randomized trial known as the Bracing in Adolescent Idiopathic Scoliosis Trial (BrAIST) demonstrated a 72% success rate at preventing curve progression to 50 degrees or more compared to 48% in the observation cohort. Given the effectiveness of bracing, the trial was terminated early. Multiple societies, including the Scoliosis Research Society (SRS), Pediatric Othopaedic Society of North America (POSNA), American Academy of Orthopaedic Surgeons (AAOS), and American Academy of Pediatrics (AAP) all recommend bracing in cases of adolescent idiopathic scoliosis with growth remaining and curves between 20-40 degrees to prevent progression and avoid surgical intervention. Needless to say, patient compliance is key: brace therapy is effective only if the brace is worn.

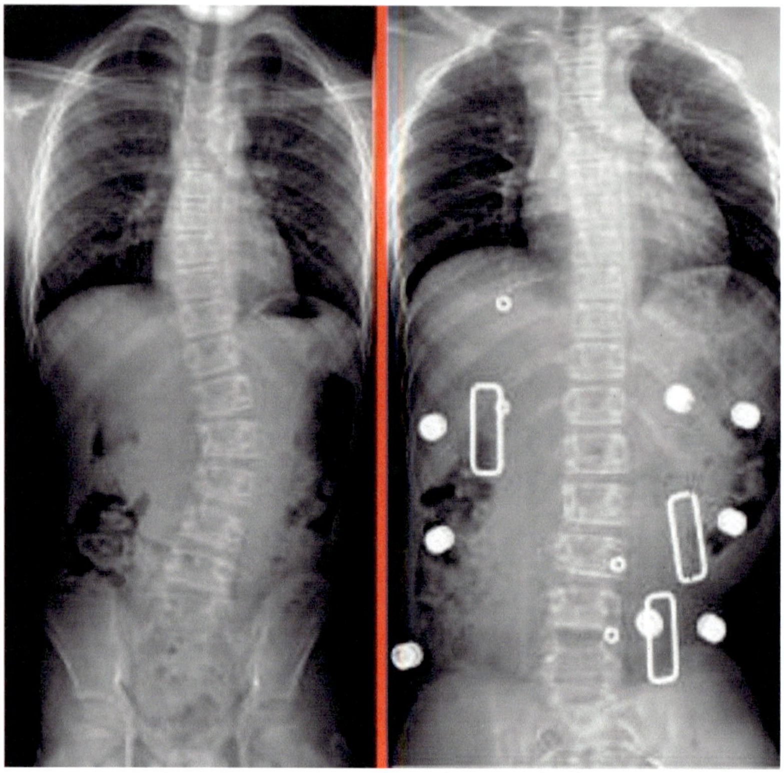

Figure 7: Anteroposterior plain film radiograph of a patient with major lumbar curve of 36 degrees prior to bracing [left] and a radiograph of the same patient in brace demonstrating curve correction while in a brace [right].

For patients with curves measuring more than 45 to 50 degrees, surgery may be the best option to correct the deformity and halt curve progression. In addition to the severity of the curve, it is ideal that patients be close to or have reached skeletal maturity.

(The precise indication for surgery is based on expert opinion. According to the website of the American Academy of Orthopaedic Surgeons in August 2020, "Most scoliosis surgeons agree that children who have very severe curves (45-50° and higher) will need surgery to lessen the curve and prevent it from getting worse.")

Surgical techniques are variable and continue to evolve with emerging technology, but the ultimate goal is to help correct deformity and achieve a solid fusion. A common technique used today is stabilization of the spine with pedicle screws and long rods until posterior spinal fusion is achieved (Figure 8).

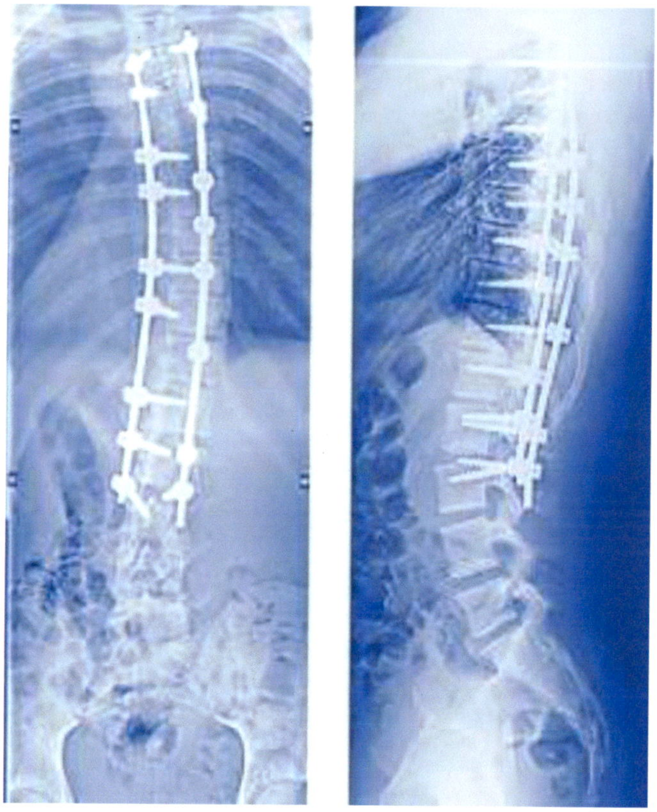

Figure 8: Surgical correction of scoliosis with a posterior spinal fusion, T4 to L3.

Surgery is usually successful. In some patients who undergo posterior spinal fusion at a young age, the anterior column of the spine can continue to grow, creating a rotation deformity. This complication can be prevented by delaying surgery until skeletal maturity or performing anterior based spinal fusions to halt growth of the anterior vertebrae.

RISK FACTORS AND PREVENTION

Currently, there are no known preventable risk factors for adolescent idiopathic scoliosis. As such, much effort has been focused on screening to help with early diagnosis and bracing to prevent the need for surgery.

A few studies have reported on the relationship with scoliosis and exercise and/or posture. Although healthy ergonomic posture and core strengthening are encouraged, there is no Level 1 evidence that demonstrates prevention or reversal of scoliosis based on posture and exercise or physical therapy programs.

Although adolescent idiopathic scoliosis is considered to be painless, residual curves (especially those measuring 50 degrees or more) may be associated with increased incidence of low back pain in adulthood.

MISCELLANY

Scoliosis need not interfere with high level athletic performance. Usain Bolt (Figure 9), one of the fastest sprinters in history, reported in his autobiography that he has scoliosis.

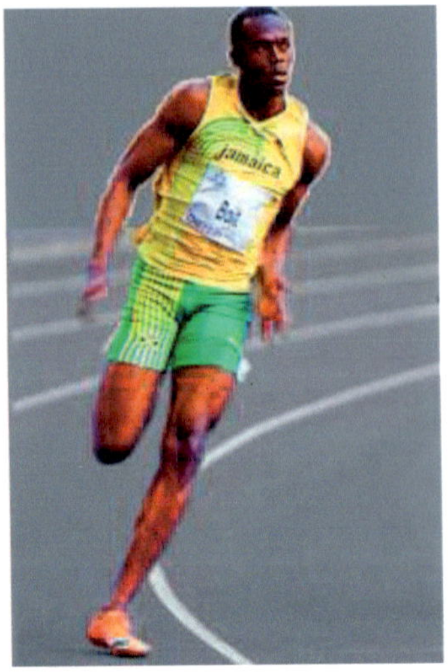

Figure 9. Usain Bolt (From Wikipedia https://commons.wikimedia.org/w/index.php?curid=7828074)

KEY TERMS

Scoliosis, Cobb angle, Risser/Sanders Assessment of Skeletal maturity, Bracing, Posterior spinal fusion

SKILLS

Define scoliosis. Be able to measure the coronal plane Cobb angle on plain film radiographs. Identify coronal and sagittal plane global balance. Recognize red flags on history and physical exam that warrant advanced imaging with MRI in patients that present with Adolescent idiopathic scoliosis. Understand criteria for bracing and surgery based on curve severity and skeletal maturity.

CHAPTER 2.

ANKYLOSING SPONDYLITIS AND OTHER SPONDYLOARTHROPATHIES

Spondyloarthropathy is a group of seronegative inflammatory rheumatic diseases of the spine. The phrase "seronegative" specifically denotes the absence of rheumatoid factor and antinuclear antibodies in the patient's circulation. The main forms of seronegative spondyloarthropathy are ankylosing spondylitis, reactive arthritis (such as Reiter's syndrome), psoriatic arthritis and spinal illnesses linked to inflammatory bowel diseases, such as Crohn's disease or ulcerative colitis.

Spondyloarthropathy is characterized by back pain and stiffness. In some cases, there are systemic manifestations affecting the eyes, gastrointestinal tract, and skin. Spondyloarthropathy is associated with joint inflammation and cartilage destruction, which leads to immobility in the musculoskeletal system. Although not detectable with routine blood tests for common antibodies, spondyloarthropathy, especially ankylosing spondylitis, is associated with a higher prevalence of the human leukocyte antigen B27 (HLA-B27) gene.

STRUCTURE AND FUNCTION

Spondyloarthropathy results in joint inflammation and cartilage destruction, which results in pain and loss of motion at the affected joint. In the spine, inflammation of the annulus surrounding the nucleus pulposus of the intervertebral disc leads to subsequent bone formation within the disc. Bone can form between the intervertebral discs too, producing so-called syndesmophytes. Ultimately, syndesmophytes can bridge one vertebral body to those adjacent to it, leading to ankyloses (fusion) of the spine.

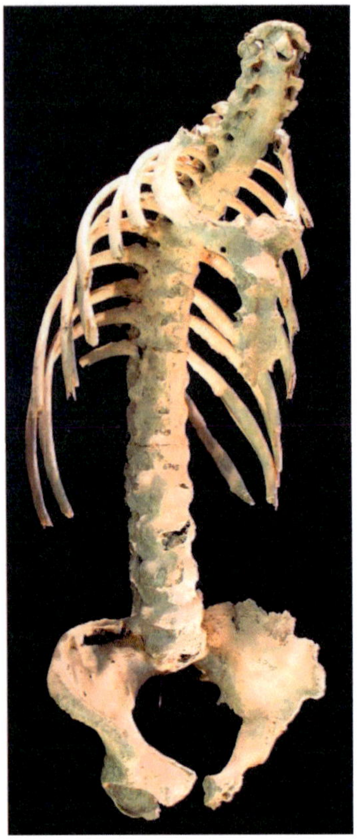

Figure 1: The spine in ankylosing spondylitis with osteophytes bridging adjoining vertebral bodies. (Courtesy of Wikipedia)

Inflammation of the attachment of the longitudinal ligaments also promotes soft-tissue ossification which contributes to the fusion of otherwise normally mobile segments. Spondyloarthropathy can induce synovitis affecting the facet joints between adjacent articular processes.

There is a strong susceptibility to spondyloarthropathy in people with the human leukocyte antigen B27 (HLA-B27) phenotype. Human leukocyte antigens are part of the major histocompatibility complex. Their function is to present antigens to cytotoxic T cells. Thus, HLA-B27 likely predisposes individuals to develop spondyloarthritis via an auto-immune reaction initiated by a response to an environmental factor or infectious pathogen. The exact mechanism, however, remains unknown.

In ankylosing spondylitis, the sacroiliac joint and the pubic symphysis are the most commonly affected joints in the body. Further inflammation leads to ascending fusion of the lumbar, thoracic and cervical vertebrae, ultimately resulting in a "bamboo spine" appearance on x-ray.

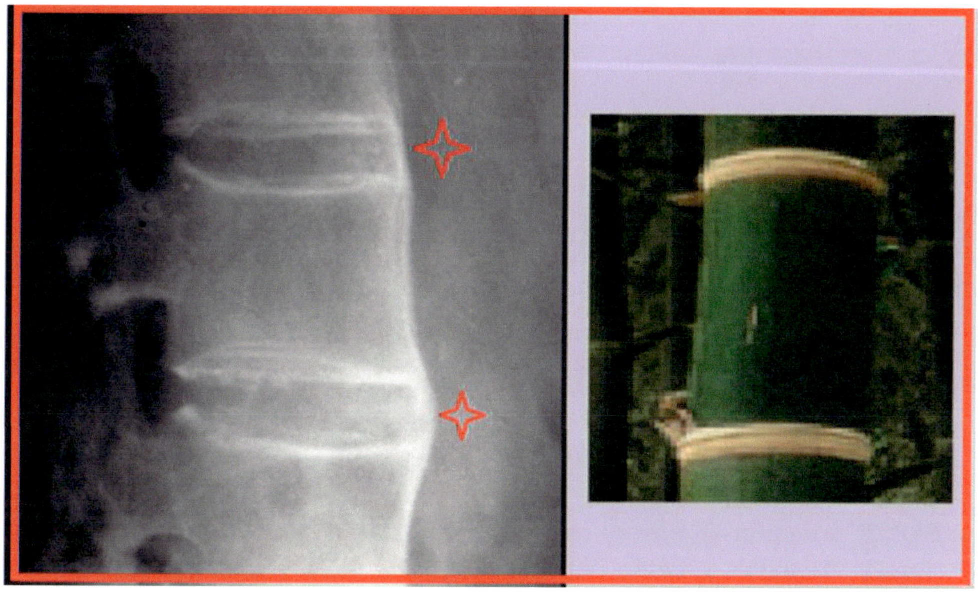

Figure 2: A radiograph showing ankylosing spondylitis with well-formed syndesmophytes, as denoted by the red stars. These osteophytes are said to resemble the culms, or rings, of bamboo, shown in the image to the right. Thus, the radiographic appearance of ankylosing spondylitis is termed "bamboo spine." (Case courtesy of Frank Gaillard, Radiopaedia.org, rID: 7163)

Reactive arthritis, as the name suggests, is thought to occur in response to an exogenous insult, such as an infection. Common pathogens include viruses and bacteria such as chlamydia, yersinia, salmonella, shigella, and campylobacter. While reactive arthritis can affect the spine, it can also commonly affect other joints of the body.

Psoriatic arthritis occurs in patients with psoriasis. In a small set of patients, the classic skin findings associated with psoriasis may be absent at the onset of joint symptoms. Nonetheless, many of these patients will eventually develop the characteristic rash.

Patients with inflammatory bowel disease often have spondyloarthropathy. In a 20-year prospective cohort study of approximately 500 patients with ulcerative colitis or Crohn's disease, ankylosing spondylitis developed in about 5% of patients, with an additional 20% reporting back pain without objective findings in the spine. Notably, the symptoms of the underlying bowel disease were reportedly worse in patients who had spondyloarthropathy compared to those who did not.

PATIENT PRESENTATION

The prototypical presentation of ankylosing spondylitis is a male in his 20s complaining of lower back pain and stiffness of insidious onset. This pain is worse in the morning and improves with activity, in contrast to osteoarthritis, which is relieved with rest and worsens with activity.

On physical exam, decreased spine motion in the anterior-posterior plane is most evident. The Schober test (Figure 3) can be used to evaluate lumbar stiffness.

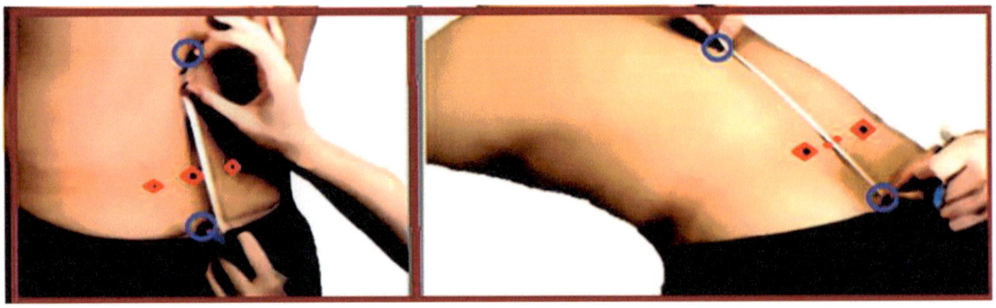

Figure 3: The Schober test is performed as follows: while standing behind the patient, the examiner identifies the line between the two iliac crests, shown here as red diamonds. The examiner then makes two marks on the skin over the lumbar spine, 15cm apart, one 5cm below the iliac line and one 10cm above it. (Both shown as blue circles). The patient is then asked to bend forward while keeping the knees straight, as if to touch the toes. The distance between the two marked points is measured again [panel at right]. If the distance of the two points does not increase by at least 5cm, lumbar stiffness is diagnosed.

Pain with the FABER maneuver (Figure 4) can help localize symptoms to the sacroiliac joint. This test is performed by placing the supine patient's hip in a position of flexion, abduction and external rotation, and having the examiner press on the flexed knee toward the pelvis, thereby loading the sacroiliac joint.

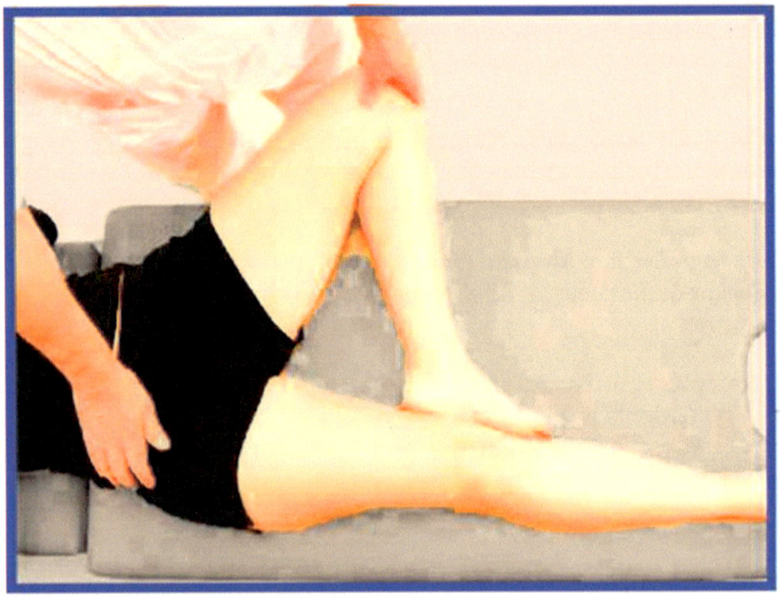

Figure 4: The FABER maneuver (courtesy study on sacroiliac joint diagnostics. Manuelle Medizin 56, 239–248 (2018). https://doi.org/10.1007/s00337-018-0405-6). Here, the examiner's left hand places a force on the patient's left SI joint. Pain localizing to the SI joint is considered a positive response.

Advanced ankylosing spondylitis is associated with a disabling thoracolumbar kyphotic deformity in more than 30% of cases. In advanced cases, ankylosis of the rib case and thoracic spine will limit chest wall expansion. Total chest wall expansion of less than 2.0 cm (normal is about 3 to 5 cm) is considered diagnostic. When chest wall expansion is limited, the patient may experience shortness of breath.

Patients with reactive arthritis classically have a triad of findings: conjunctivitis, urethritis and arthritis. (Arthritis often occurs later in the course than the other two symptoms.) In many cases, patients can recall a history of recent viral or bacterial infection 1 to 3 weeks prior to the onset of symptoms.

A distinctive feature of reactive arthritis is dactylitis, in which one or two fingers or toes becomes diffusely swollen. A small fraction of patients (< 10%) present with cardiac manifestations of the disease, such as aortic regurgitation or pericarditis.

Psoriatic arthritis most commonly affects the limbs, but in about 40% of cases, the cervical spine or the sacroiliac joint can be affected. Most of the patients have a history of psoriatic rash (Figure 5) prior to the appearance of arthritis, some develop the rash and arthritis concurrently and others present with arthritis first.

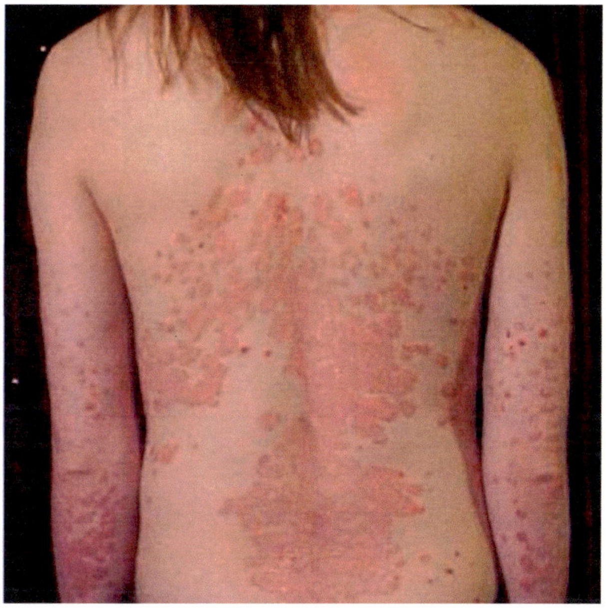

Figure 5. Skin manifestation of psoriasis. (Courtesy Wikipedia)

Enthesopathies involving the Achilles tendon, patellar tendon and plantar fascia are often seen.

Extra-articular manifestations are common with spondyloarthropathies. Uveitis (Figure 6) is the most frequent extra-articular manifestation of ankylosing spondylitis, occurring in ~25% of patients. This manifests as acute unilateral eye pain, blurred vision, photophobia and lachrymation (increased tear production).

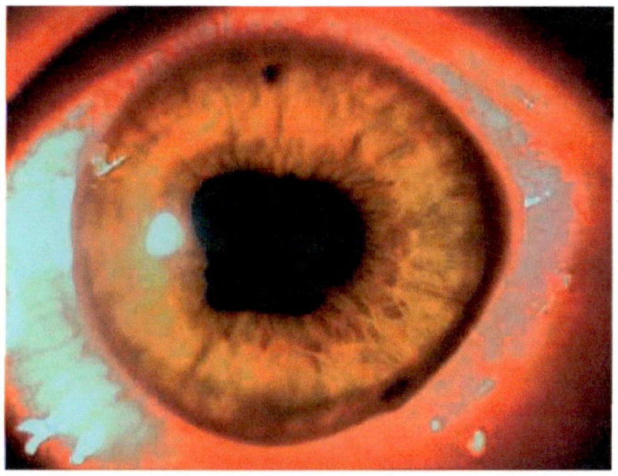

Figure 6: Chronic anterior uveitis with dilated conjunctival blood vessels and deformed pupil due to anterior synechiae (adhesions of the iris). (Courtesy of Ocular manifestations of rheumatic diseases. Int Ophthalmol 40, 503–510 (2020). https://doi.org/10.1007/s10792-019-01183-9)

OBJECTIVE EVIDENCE

Laboratory findings

There are no specific serological tests for seronegative spondyloarthropathies. Elevation of the erythrocyte sedimentation rate (ESR) or C-reactive protein (CRP) levels are suggestive of inflammation, but are nonspecific. The tests for rheumatoid factor (RF) and anti-nuclear antibody (ANA) are, by definition, normal in seronegative spondyloarthropathy. The synovial fluid may also show an increased preponderance of white blood cells, particularly neutrophils, but this finding is also nonspecific.

While there is a strong correlation to the HLA-B27 gene, only a scant minority (1-2%) of those with the HLA-B27 gene ever develop spondyloarthropathies. The prevalence of the HLA-B27 gene varies by race, ethnicity and geographic location. In the United States, the estimated prevalence is about 7% among Caucasians but less than 1% among African Americans. Only 10% of patients with spondyloarthropathies test negative for the HLA-B27 gene. Taken together, testing for the HLA-B27 gene is neither sensitive nor specific enough to make a definitive diagnosis.

Radiographic findings

In patients with suspected ankylosing spondylitis, full-length AP and lateral plain radiographs of the spine and pelvis should be obtained.

Sacroiliac erosions and joint space changes are characteristic and are the first radiographic features observed (Figure 7).

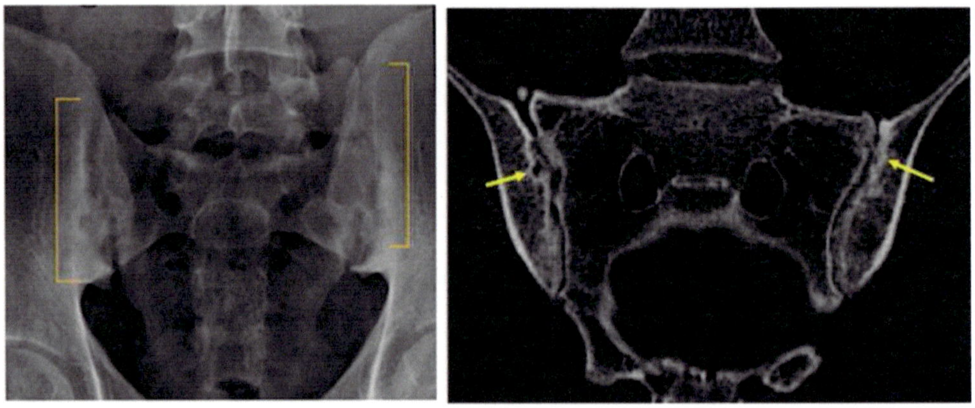

Figure 7: Inflammation with widening of the sacroiliac joints (sacroiliitis) is seen bilaterally in the panel to the left (Case courtesy of Dr Mark Holland, Radiopaedia.org, rID: 23359); on the right, a CT scan shows sacroiliac joint erosion with regional sclerosis of subchondral bone (Case courtesy of Lukas, Cédric et al. RMD open vol. 4,1 e000586. 12 Jan. 2018, doi:10.1136/rmdopen-2017-000586)

Another common finding is the presence of syndesmophytes that connect the vertebral bodies (as shown above).

MRI is the best modality for early detection of ankylosing spondylitis, as it can detect inflammation around the sacroiliac joints on the T2-weighted images.

EPIDEMIOLOGY

The prevalence of the spondyloarthropathies varies widely by disease type, patient race and geography.

Ankylosing spondylitis affects males approximately 3 to 4 times more frequently than it affects females. The typical age of onset is adulthood. The HLA-B27 gene is present in ~90% of patients. Overall, about 0.2% of patients in the USA are affected.

Reactive arthritis is slightly less prevalent than ankylosing spondylitis: approximately 0.1% in the US are affected. As with ankylosing spondylitis, male patients make up the majority of cases of reactive arthritis, and the typical age of onset is also in early adulthood. The HLA-B27 gene is present in ~80% of patients.

Psoriatic arthritis is found in about 0.3% of Americans. Unlike ankylosing spondylitis and reactive arthritis, psoriatic arthritis has a later age of onset (about 40 years of age) and an equal distribution among males and females.

As noted above, about 25% of patients with inflammatory bowel disease will have some form of spondyloarthropathy, but most cases do not feature sacroiliac erosions or ankylosis.

DIFFERENTIAL DIAGNOSIS

As most of the spondyloarthropathies affect younger patients, traumatic injuries should be ruled out initially. Aside from trauma which can be gleaned from a thorough history, there are other causes of non-traumatic injuries that may present in a similar manner to seronegative spondyloarthropathies.

While rare in young patients, osteoarthritis may be present, especially in the context of repetitive trauma, overuse or genetic predisposition. The defining features that help identify osteoarthritis are radiographic findings consistent with joint space narrowing, osteophyte formation, bony sclerosis, back pain that worsens as the day progresses, and the lack of inflammatory markers on blood testing.

Rheumatoid arthritis is much more common than seronegative spondyloarthropathies and thus when inflammatory markers on blood testing are elevated and the patient's back pain improves as the day progresses, rheumatoid arthritis must be considered. Notably, rheumatoid arthritis in the limbs is commonly symmetric, whereas peripheral joint involvement in spondyloarthropathies is often asymmetric. Most importantly, patients with spondyloarthropathy will test negative for rheumatoid factor and anti-nuclear antibody.

Diffuse Idiopathic Skeletal Hyperostosis ("DISH") is also a condition that can cause enthesophytes and markedly decreased range of motion of the spine. This can be differentiated from ankylosing spondylitis by the location and shape of the bony outgrowths on radiographs. Syndesmophytes are bony fusions within the joint space itself, while enthesophytes occur outside the annulus fibrosus (Figure 8). Another key distinction is that DISH has no sacroiliac joint involvement and is a disease of older men; DISH is rarely seen in patients younger than 50 years of age.

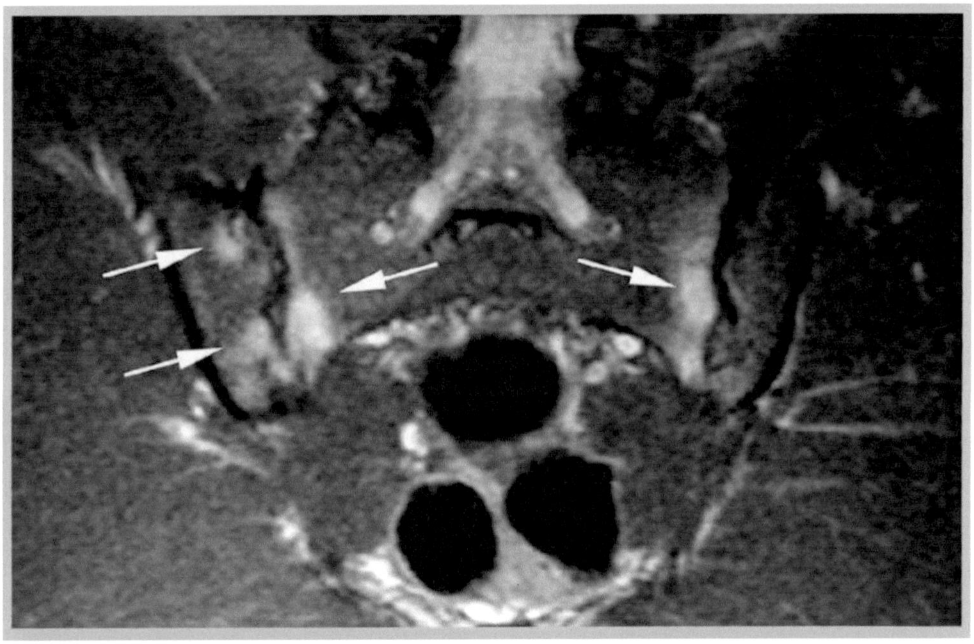

Figure 8: T2-weighted coronal MRI image with fat signal saturation, showing bone marrow edema in the upper and middle thirds of sacroiliac joints (arrows). (Image courtesy of Rev. Bras. Reumatol. 57 (5) Sep-Oct 2017, https://doi.org/10.1016/j.rbre.2016.09.002)

RED FLAGS

The most concerning spondyloarthropathy is ankylosing spondylitis, as it can severely reduce the patient's life expectancy and quality of life. Restriction of chest wall movement, decreased mobility, and heightened susceptibility to fracture after even minor trauma are the major sources of morbidity and mortality. (Reactive arthritis and psoriatic arthritis, while painful, usually do not affect the patient's life expectancy.) Thus, when a young man with no history of trauma presents with insidious lower back pain, ankylosing spondylitis must not be missed. The red flags suggesting ankylosing spondylitis include lower back pain in a young patient with no history of recent trauma or repetitive stress, symptoms that improve during the day or with activity, and the gradual migration of the pain from the lumbosacral region to the neck over time. In addition, radiographs of the pelvis have the characteristic pattern of sacroiliac joint fusion.

Among patients with known spondyloarthropathy, the syndesmophytes present render the spine brittle and minimally compliant. Thus, patients with ankylosing spondylitis are highly susceptible to unstable spine fractures and neurologic injury with low energy trauma. Diagnostic vigilance and a high index of suspicion for fracture must be maintained when evaluating a patient with known ankylosing spondylitis after trauma. CT and/or MRI are needed and the patient should be immobilized in their preinjury alignment pending diagnosis and treatment. Acute neck pain in a patient with long-standing ankylosing spondylitis should be immobilized and evaluated with more advanced imaging such as CT and MRI scans to exclude a fracture, even without a history of severe trauma.

TREATMENT OPTIONS AND OUTCOMES

Treatment for spondyloarthropathies begins with traditional NSAIDs or COX-2 inhibitors. Physical therapy can also be prescribed to maintain mobility and reduce pain. NSAIDs should be taken with caution in patients with spondyloarthropathy associated inflammatory bowel disease.

Seronegative spondyloarthropathies, in general, are chronic and insidious diseases. Reactive arthritis may be the exception, as most cases are either self-limited or relapsing-remitting. The majority of reactive arthritis patients have severe symptoms lasting weeks to months that eventually disappear. However, about 15% of patients may develop chronic or progressive arthritis.

For patients who do not respond sufficiently to NSAIDs/COX-2 inhibitors (or for those who have complications compelling their cessation), biological response modifiers and disease-modifying antirheumatic drugs (DMARDs) may be considered. Biological response modifiers aim to block the interaction between inflammatory cells and include agents such as infliximab or etanercept, which are TNF-alpha inhibitors, or IL-12 inhibitors. DMARDs include methotrexate, cyclosporine, azathioprine, and sulfasalazine. DMARDs produce their immunosuppressive effects by suppressing the growth and maturation of inflammatory cells.

Debilitating kyphotic deformities in ankylosing spondylitis can be treated with an osteotomy and fusion (Figure 9).

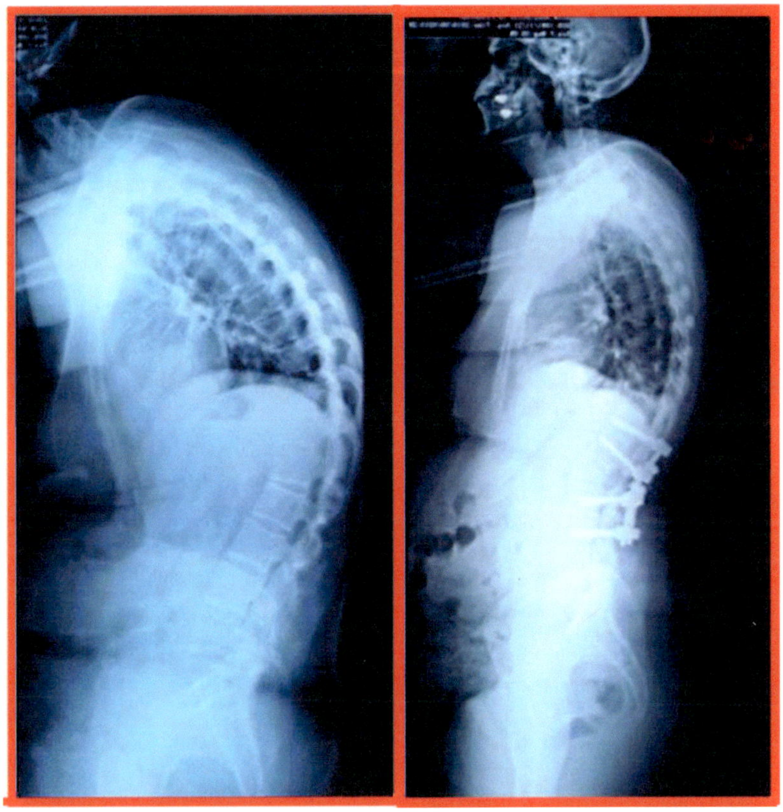

Figure 9: Kyphosis in ankylosing spondylitis is decreased from 72 degrees preoperatively (left) to 25 degrees (right) with a mini-open pedicle subtraction osteotomy. (Courtesy of BMC Musculoskeletal Disorders 22, 101 (2021). https://doi.org/10.1186/s12891-021-03974-7)

Patients with advanced spondyloarthropathies are at risk for spinal fractures, most commonly in the mid-cervical or the cervicothoracic junction or lower at the thoracolumbar junction. While stable fractures with no accompanying epidural hemorrhage can be treated with traction or halo immobilization devices alone, instability, hemorrhage and neurological changes suggest a need for surgical intervention. The most common technique involves decompression at the site of injury to remove the hematoma, followed by spinal fusion to stabilize the area. In some cases, osteotomies are necessary to correct severe kyphotic deformities.

RISK FACTORS AND PREVENTION

Spondyloarthropathy is a risk factor for spinal fracture and spinal cord injury. Indeed, the incidence of spinal cord injury among patients with ankylosing spondylitis is more than 10 times greater than that of the general population.

There are no known preventive measures for seronegative spondyloarthropathies. Although viral or bacterial infections are associated with reactive arthritis in HLA-B27 positive patients, any small infection may lead to the development of arthritis, making it difficult to prevent.

It is particularly important that patients with spondyloarthropathy, especially ankylosing spondylitis, stop smoking. The disease itself can cause shortness of breath, in addition to the dyspnea that smoking may cause.

For patients with spondyloarthropathy, exercises that focus on increasing flexibility with low impact such Pilates or Tai Chi may improve function.

KEY TERMS

Seronegative spondyloarthropathy, ankylosing spondylitis, reactive arthritis, bamboo-spine

SKILLS

Perform a comprehensive history and physical exam in patients presenting with back pain. Recognize the x-ray findings in spondyloarthropathy.

CHAPTER 3.

BURNERS AND STINGERS

DESCRIPTION

A burner or stinger is characterized by brief, unilateral arm pain, paresthesias or weakness after an injury or a specific inciting event. A burner or stinger is caused by a transient brachial plexus injury (so-called neuropraxia) due to traction, compression, or direct trauma to the brachial plexus. It is often associated with collision sports injuries, such as football, that causes bending of the neck and/or displacement of the arm. Treatment is usually not necessary, and players can return to play when and if there is complete resolution of symptoms.

STRUCTURE AND FUNCTION

The brachial plexus comprises of nerve roots from C5-T1 (Figure 1). There are five regions to the brachial plexus from proximal to distal: Roots, Trunks, Divisions, Cords, Branches.

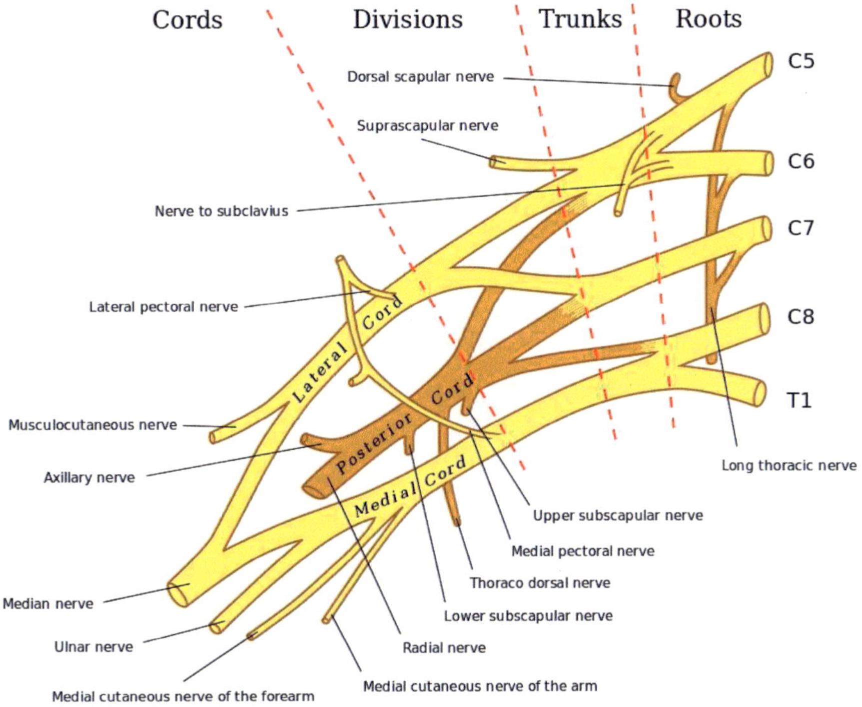

Figure 1: A "wiring diagram" of the brachial plexus. (from https://en.wikipedia.org/wiki/Brachial_plexus)

Roots – The nerve roots are composed of the ventral and dorsal components, each carrying motor and sensory information, respectively. The two combine to form the cervical nerve roots and exit the spine. The 5 cervical roots combine to form 3 trunks.

Trunks – The superior (C5, C6), middle (C7), and inferior (C8, T1) trunks emerge between the anatomical triangle formed by the anterior scalene muscle, middle scalene muscle, and the first rib. After traversing a short distance, each trunk divides into anterior and posterior divisions.

Divisions – There are six divisions (3 anterior, 3 posterior) that combine into 3 cords, which now have different coverage from the C5-T1 roots compared to the 3 trunks.

Cords – The posterior cord (C5-C8) is formed from the 3 posterior divisions. Prior to the final branches, the posterior cord gives off the upper subscapular nerve (C5, C6; innervates subscapularis), the lower subscapular nerve (C5, C6; innervates subscapularis and teres major), and the thoracodorsal nerve (C6-C8; innervates latissimus dorsi).

The lateral cord (C5-C7) is formed from the anterior divisions of the superior and middle trunks. Prior to its final branching, it gives off the lateral pectoral nerve (C5-C7; innervates pectoralis major).

The medial cord (C8, T1) is formed from the anterior division of the inferior trunk. Prior to its final branching, it gives off the medial pectoral nerve (C8, T1; innervates pectoralis minor and major), the medial brachial cutaneous nerve (T1), and the medial antebrachial cutaneous nerve (C8, T1). Each cord gives off two terminal branches.

Branches – There are five terminal branches (two branches form the median nerve).

1. The axillary nerve (C5, C6) derives from the posterior cord and travels to the glenohumeral joint. It mainly innervates the deltoid as well as sensation to the lateral shoulder.
2. The radial nerve (C5-T1) derives from the posterior cord and runs medially along the arm with the long head of the triceps until it crosses laterally across the humerus via the spiral groove. The nerve supplies the elbow and forearm extensors and supinators. The nerve also provides sensation to the distal-lateral arm, the posterior forearm, and the posterior aspect of the radial side of the hand (thumb to middle finger).
3. The median nerve (C5-C7) derives from the medial and the lateral cord. The cords join anterior to the axillary artery and then travels with the artery along the arm. The nerve innervates most wrist flexors and pronators as well as the two lumbricals on the radial side of the hand. The nerve provides sensation to the anterior aspect of the radial side of the hand.
4. The musculocutaneous nerve (C5-C7) derives from the medial cord and pierces through the coracobrachialis muscle to become the most superficial branch. The nerve innervates the biceps, coracobrachialis, and brachialis. The nerve provides sensation to the lateral forearm.
5. The ulnar nerve (C8, T1) derives from the medial cord and runs along the medial aspect of the arm, through the cubital tunnel at the elbow and through Guyon's canal at the wrist. The nerve innervates the flexor carpi ulnaris, the adductor pollicis, and the intrinsic hand muscles (except the two radial lumbricals innervated by the median nerve). The nerve provides sensation to the whole ulnar aspect of the hand.

Most cases of stingers affect the C5/C6 nerve roots or the upper trunk of the plexus.

The most common cause of injury is due to traction on the brachial plexus rather than direct trauma. This can occur in ipsilateral shoulder depression and neck deviation towards the contralateral side, often seen in tackling, which causes stretching of the brachial plexus on the ipsilateral side.

PATIENT PRESENTATION

Most athletes present after particularly high-impact collisions, with immediate onset of unilateral, radiating, and severe burning pain down the arm. This may be accompanied by paresthesia in the related sensory dermatome (the area of skin sensation supplied by a given spinal nerve) and motor weakness. Players may be supporting the affected arm using the other arm to relieve tension. Neck pain is usually not present.

On physical exam, transient sensory disturbances (numbness, tingling, burning, or radiating pain) in the affected arm are common (Figure 2). There may be transient, unilateral weakness in the affected arm with normal biceps reflexes (Figure 3 – Figure 7). (Transient hyporeflexia may be present in a minority of patients).

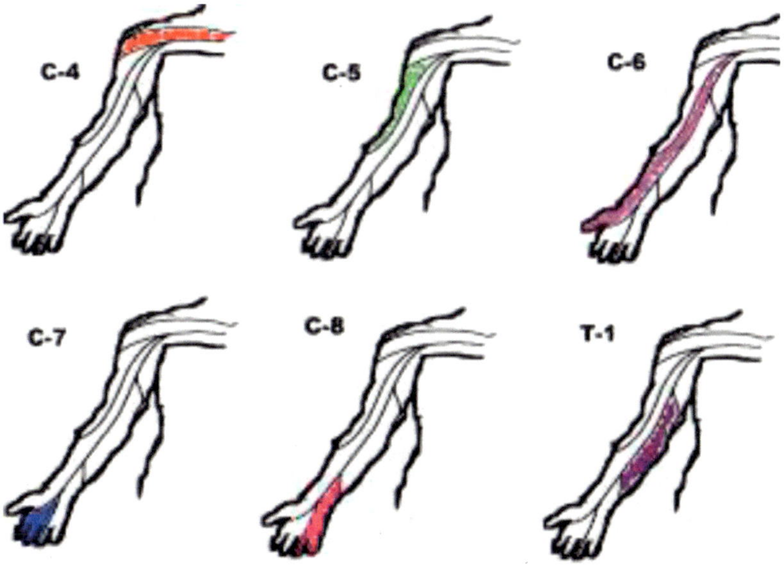

Figure 2: The sensory dermatomes as shown on the volar (palmar) side of the arm. Lesions at the given level would be expected to produce sensory changes in these locations, if any.

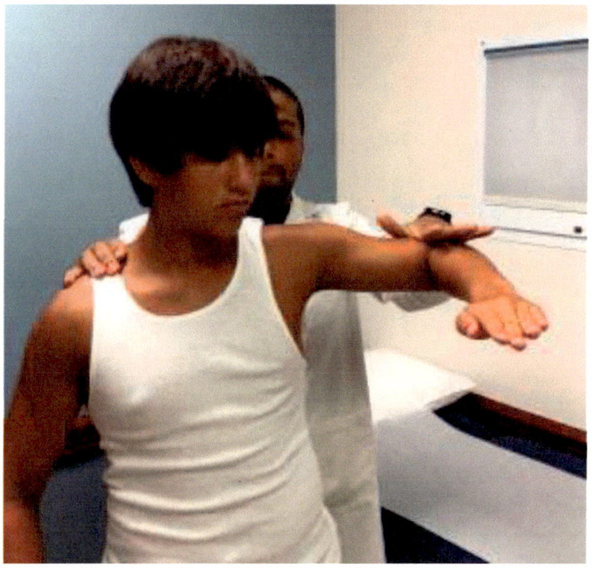

Figure 3: C-5 Motor exam: assessing shoulder abduction. With the elbow flexed, the patient abducts the shoulder to 90. The examiner pushes down on the elbow as the patient resists with deltoid activity.

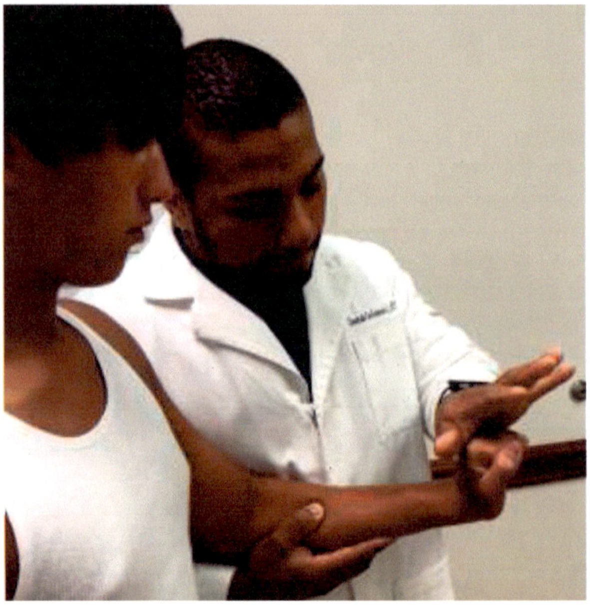

Figure 4: The C-6 Motor exam: assessing wrist extension. With the forearm pronated, the patient extends the wrist. The examiner can assess strength by pushing down on the knuckle of the index finger as the patient resists with radial wrist extensor activity.

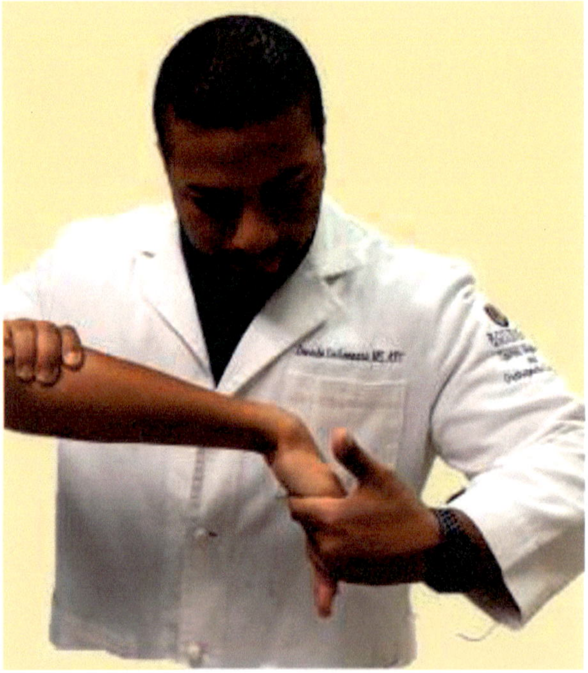

Figure 5: The C-7 Motor exam: assessing wrist flexion. With fingers extended, the patient flexes the wrist. The examiner pushes against the palm to force the wrist into extension as the patient resists. (As with the C-6 exam, the patient's fingers are positioned to eliminate the indirect effect of finger muscles on wrist motion.)

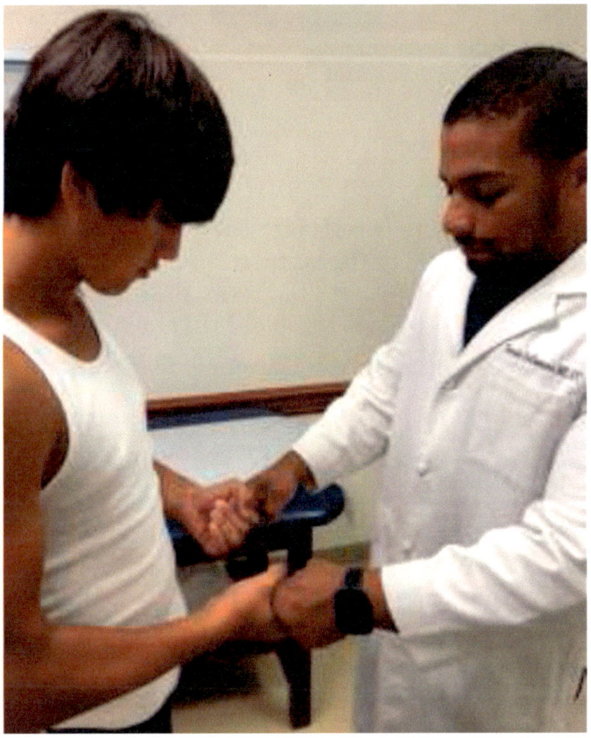

Figure 6: The C-8 Motor exam: assessing finger flexion/grip strength. Have the patient attempt to squeeze the examiner's index and long finger simultaneously.

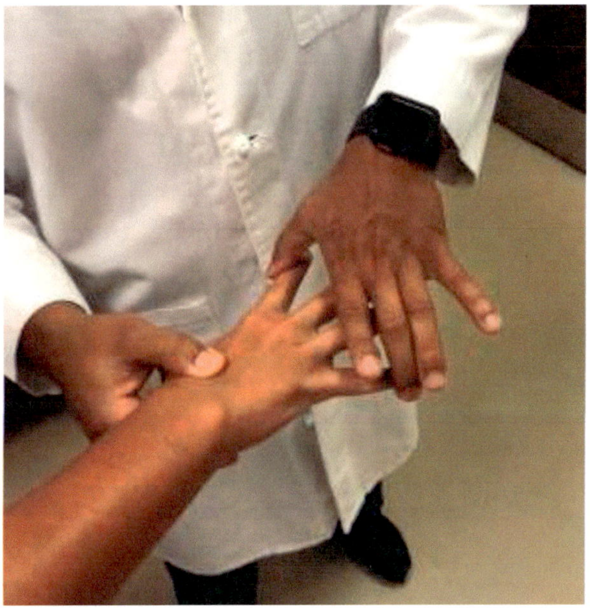

Figure 7: The T-1 Motor examination: assessing finger abduction. Ask the patient to spread (abduct) the fingers and hold that position; the examiner can assess strength by attempting to resist this as shown.The lower extremity exam should be normal, and if it is not, the diagnosis of a stinger is questioned.

The key finding is that these symptoms, if present, should be transient. The vast majority of cases resolve within a few minutes to days.

All cases of stingers can be classified into 3 grades. Grade 1 stingers are due to neuropraxia (intact axon but demyelinated). There may be temporary loss of sensation and/or motor function up to days. Grade 2 stingers are due to axonotmesis (axon damage). This produces more significant motor and/or sensory deficits which may last up to several weeks. Last, Grade 3 stingers are due to neurotmesis (severed nerves). This may produce enduring symptoms that may never fully resolve.

OBJECTIVE EVIDENCE

In most cases of first-time stingers, imaging is not necessary. Initial imaging, if obtained, usually consists of anterior-posterior, lateral, and oblique views of the cervical spine and shoulder area. No abnormal findings are found in most cases of simple stingers. If there are concerns for further pathology due to Red Flag findings mentioned below, and if initial imaging is normal, cervical MRI should be obtained to evaluate the spinal cord, nerve roots, vertebral discs, ligamentous injury, or vertebral fractures.

There are no specific laboratory findings associated with stingers or other cervical spine diseases.

EPIDEMIOLOGY

Stingers are most commonly seen in football players, but can also be seen in hockey, lacrosse, and rugby players. This is because the mechanism of injury is usually forced rapid lateral neck flexion, which can occur during tackling and can cause traction or compression injuries to the brachial plexus. It is estimated that over 50% of football players have reported at least one stinger during their career. The true prevalence of this condition is not known, mainly due to its transient nature and the tendency of players to not report or underreport their symptoms.

DIFFERENTIAL DIAGNOSIS

The differential diagnosis for stingers is relatively narrow but should be considered in any cases when red flags (as discussed below) are present.

- Cervical radiculopathy: Consider if symptoms persist beyond 24 hours. MRI can help assess for radiculopathy. Presentation may be similar to burners and stingers, other than the timeframe of symptoms.
- Shoulder dislocation or acromioclavicular joint injury: Injury to the bony structures of the shoulder should be considered, especially after traumatic sports injuries affecting one arm. X-rays, CT, or MRI can help assess for injuries to the bones or surrounding soft tissue.
- Thoracic outlet syndrome: This syndrome is thought to be caused by compression of the brachial plexus or subclavian vessels as they pass through narrow passageways leading from the base of the neck and torso out to the arm (the "thoracic outlet"). This compression can cause neck and arm pain and paresthesias in the fingers and hand. At times, the affected hand is pale and cool. Thoracic outlet syndrome seems to be provoked by rotation of the head and neck.
- Cervical spine stenosis or fracture: In severe cases of collision, the actual spinal canal may be damaged. If this is the case, players may present with bilateral symptoms or have symptoms in their lower extremities, which never occurs with stingers. The cervical spine should be immobilized until further evaluation by CT or MRI.

RED FLAGS

If any of the following signs are present in a patient presenting for stingers, further workup should be considered to rule out the above differential diagnoses.

- Bilateral symptoms: Stingers affect only one arm at a time. Bilateral symptoms should raise concern for spinal canal stenosis or cervical fractures.
- Lower extremity symptoms: Stingers affect only the brachial plexus. Lower extremity symptoms should raise concern for spinal cord injuries.
- Muscle atrophy: Stingers, due to their transient nature, rarely causes atrophy. If significant atrophy is present, consider recurrent stingers or other pathologies.
- Symptoms lasting more than 24 hours: While stingers can last longer than 24 hours, the majority of cases last under 24 hours. Further imaging should be pursued if symptoms last for over 24 hours to rule out more dangerous pathologies, covered above.

TREATMENT OPTIONS AND OUTCOMES

The most important step in treating suspected stingers is to remove the player from play for initial evaluation. A quick but thorough exam of all four extremities as well as the neck should be conducted to assess for findings and red flags discussed in this chapter. A player may return to play upon complete resolution of symptoms and once he/she demonstrates normal strength and range of motion of the affected arm. Recurring or persistent symptoms should be evaluated as discussed earlier. If symptoms last for more than a few minutes, cervical x-rays should be strongly considered to evaluate for fractures or dislocations.

For persistent symptoms, after appropriate work up showing no other pathology, rest and gentle stretching of the affected arm is advised. Physical therapy may be recommended if symptoms persist beyond a few days. Specific stretching and posturing maneuvers can be recommended by the therapist. NSAIDs may be used to alleviate pain during the first few days.

Surgery is almost never considered for stingers. In rare cases of Grade 3 stingers, due to complete transection of axons, surgery may be attempted to repair the damaged axons, but outcomes are poor.

Considering that stingers rarely lead to permanent disability, the general prognosis of first-time stingers is excellent. An estimated 85% players are able to return to play within the same game or practice. A history of a prior stinger can increase the incidence of recurrent stingers, but there is no clear evidence of recurrent stingers causing permanent nerve injury.

RISK FACTORS AND PREVENTION

The most significant risk factor for the development of stingers is playing contact sports that involve tackling. The majority of such players encounter at least one episode of stingers during their career. The presence of cervical canal stenosis has been associated with increased risk of stingers in athletes.

Prevention efforts should focus on proper tackling techniques and protective equipment. A more upright tackling position may protect the neck from excessive extension, while increased padding and/or cervical collar may help absorb some of the impact.

MISCELLANY

The five sections of the brachial plexus, in order from proximal to distal (roots, trunks, divisions, cords, branches), can be memorized by the following mnemonic (Randy Travis Drinks Cold Beer).

The three terminal branches that form the famous M of the brachial plexus, in order from lateral to medial (musculocutaneous, median, ulnar), can be recalled by thinking MuMU (μ, M in Greek).

KEY TERMS

Cervical spine, brachial plexus, stingers/burners, sensory dermatome

SKILLS

Draw a "wiring diagram" of the brachial plexus from memory. (It's always on the test!) Perform a comprehensive physical exam to evaluate neurologic signs and symptoms. Counsel players on safe sports techniques and appropriate equipment to reduce future recurrences.

CHAPTER 4.

CERVICAL RADICULOPATHY AND MYELOPATHY

Both the spinal cord itself and the exiting nerve roots are subject to compression in the cervical spine. Compression neuropathy of the nerve roots is termed radiculopathy; pressure on the cord can produce myelopathy.

Radiculopathy can be caused by chronic overgrowth of the bone and soft tissue or acute disc herniation. Cervical radiculopathy presents as unilateral arm pain, paresthesias, or weakness in the areas innervated by the compressed nerve.

Myelopathy is usually caused by degenerative cervical spondylosis. Myelopathy presents in older patients as bilateral paresthesias, loss of dexterity, and impaired gait. Myelopathy can also be acute due to a large central disc herniation that compresses the spinal cord. Traumatic injuries to the cervical spine that result in bony or soft tissue compression of the cervical spinal cord can also cause myelopathy.

STRUCTURE AND FUNCTION

The spinal cord exits the cranium through the foramen magnum to enter the spinal canal. In the cervical spine, branches off the cord form the cervical nerve roots and exit through their neural foramina. The remaining cord passes to the thoracic and lumbar regions.

The cervical canal is normally about 17 mm in diameter, but varies by individual. Thus, the amount of space for the neural elements is best considered in relative terms: the ratio of the sagittal diameter of the canal to the corresponding measurement of the vertebral body. This is known as the Torg-Pavlov ratio and is usually equal to 1 (Figure 1).

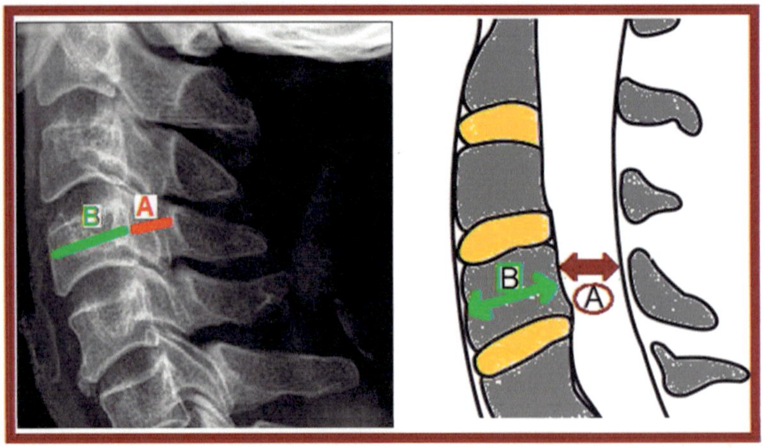

Figure 1: To calculate the Torg-Pavlov ratio, the sagittal diameter of the spinal canal (A) is measured from the posterior surface of the vertebral body to the nearest point of the corresponding spinal laminar line. The sagittal diameter of the vertebral body (B) is measured at the midpoint between the anterior surface and the posterior surface. The Torg-Pavlov ratio is A/B. (The drawing and radiograph are modified from Clin Orthop Surg. 2009 Mar; 1(1) via creative commons license.)

The spinal cord takes up an increasing fraction of the spinal canal moving distally: the cord takes about 50% of the space at C1, but about 75% at C6. Narrowing of the canal, or stenosis, can lead to compression of the spinal cord and symptoms of myelopathy.

The most common cause of cervical stenosis and resulting myelopathy is age-related degenerative change. Degenerative change includes protrusion of the discs, hypertrophy of the ligaments and osseous overgrowth. Degenerative change can also produce a slippage of one vertebral body over the other (spondylolisthesis) which can compress the cord as well. Degenerative changes are most frequently seen at C5, C6 and C7.

Congenital stenosis is also possible, although much less common. Rheumatoid arthritis, producing both synovial overgrowth as well as slippage from facet arthritis, might also reduce the amount of space available for the spinal cord.

At each cervical level, dorsal (sensory) and ventral (motor) neurons combine to form nerve roots. These roots exit the spine through the lateral neural foramen. It is important to keep in mind, that in the cervical spine, each named nerve root exits *above* the corresponding vertebral pedicle, that is, the C6 nerve root exits between C5 and C6 (Figure 2) whereas in the thoracic and lumbar spine, the nerve roots exit *below* the corresponding pedicle (i.e. the L2 nerve root exits between L2 and L3). The C8 nerve root exits between C7 and T1 to allow for this transition.

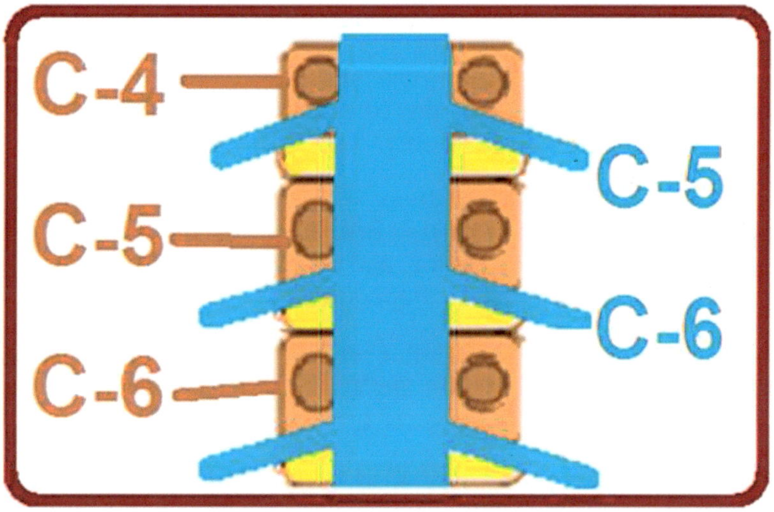

Figure 2: The cervical nerve roots are shown and labeled in blue, and the vertebral bodies are shown and labeled in brown. As noted, the C-6 root exits above the C6 vertebral body.

The cervical nerve roots travel from the cord in a *horizontal* orientation, whereas lumbar nerve roots travel distally with *vertical* orientation before moving laterally. Thus, in the cervical spine, both centrally-located and peripheral masses will compress the same nerve root. By contrast, in the lumbar spine, a lateral or foraminal mass will compress the nerve root on the verge of exit, whereas a central or paracentral disc herniation will compress the nerve root that is traveling distally to exit one level lower (the traversing nerve root).

The distinctions between cervical and lumbar nerve herniations based on central vs lateral location is demonstrated in Figure 3.

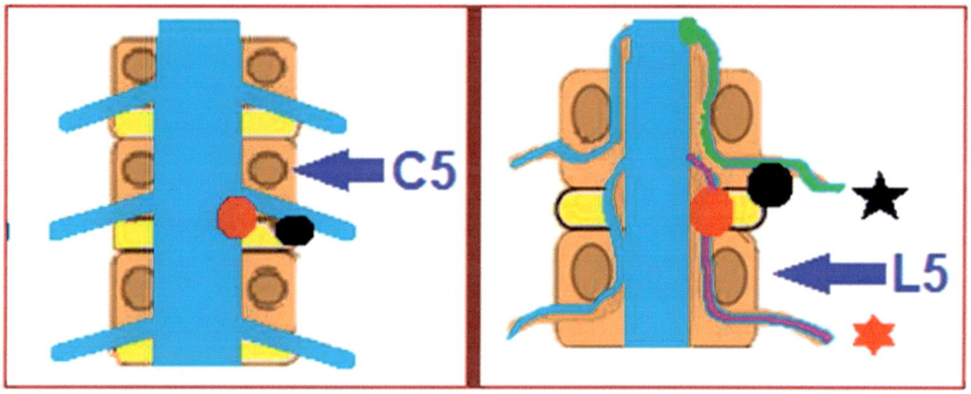

Figure 3: The cervical nerve roots, left panel, diverge from the spinal cord horizontally, such that a central disc herniation (shown as a red circle) and a lateral disc herniation (black circle) compress the same nerve root: i.e., a C 5/6 disc herniation compresses the C6 root, as shown, independent of how lateral the disc herniation might be. On the other hand, in the lumbar spine (shown at right) the nerve root travels distally in a vertical orientation close to the cord for approximately one vertebral level. Thus, a central disc herniation of the L 4/5 disc (shown in red) will compress the traversing L5 nerve root that is still central (the L5 root is shown in purple, terminating at the red star), yet a lateral disc herniation at this level (black circle) will compress the exiting L4 root (shown in green, terminating at the black star).

PATIENT PRESENTATION

Cervical spine stenosis is often asymptomatic. Also, myelopathy and radiculopathy are not exclusive: a combined condition termed myeloradiculopathy due to age-related degenerative changes can be present. The entire clinical picture–history, physical, and diagnostic imaging–must be considered.

Myelopathy first presents with neck pain or stiffness. There is extremity numbness and tingling in a non-dermatomal distribution, usually bilaterally, affecting first the upper and then the lower extremities. There is motor weakness, difficulty with fine motor function, and decreased coordination; there may be gait instability and urinary incontinence with more progressive compression.

The neurologic exam will reveal weakness (though this can be subtle) and decreased ability for rapid, repetitive movements. Abnormal proprioception (as seen on the "finger to nose with eyes closed" test) may be present. Additional findings include hyperreflexia and impaired heel-toe walking.

Cord compression may be suggested by two special signs: the Hoffmann sign and the Babinski reflex. The Hoffman sign (Figure 4) is noted when there is involuntary flexion or adduction of the thumb when the examiner flicks the fingernail of the middle finger down. Babinski's sign (Figure 5) is seen when the great toe extends involuntarily in response to the examiner's scratching the outer underside of the patient's foot. The normal response is for the toes to curl downwards. (Babinski's sign is also present in normal babies under the age of 2 months.)

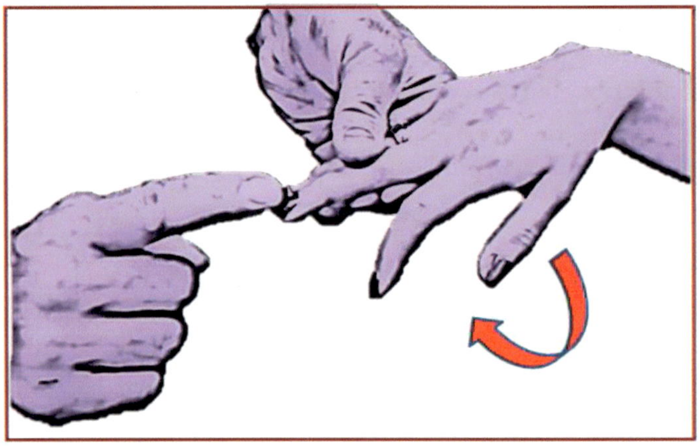

Figure 4: Hoffman sign is seen when the thumb involuntarily adducts or flexes in response to the examiner's flicking of the middle finger.

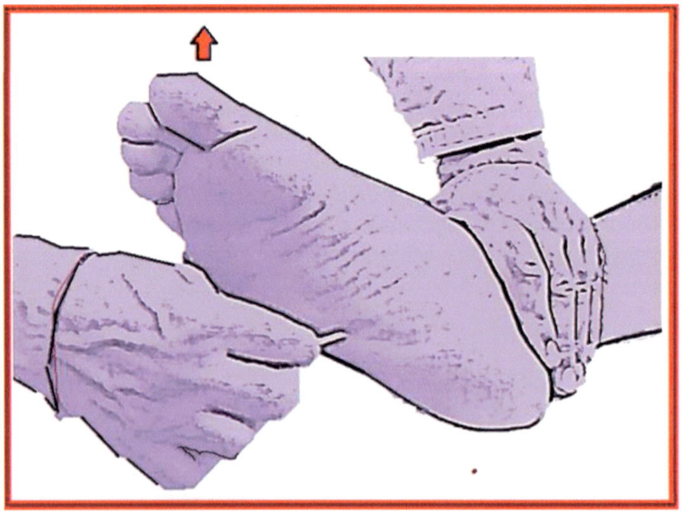

Figure 5: Babinski's sign is observed when the great toe extends involuntarily in response to the examiner's scratching the outer underside of the patient's foot.

Radiculopathy may also present with neck pain or stiffness, but the characteristic finding is pain and paresthesias in a dermatomal distribution in the arm (Figure 6).

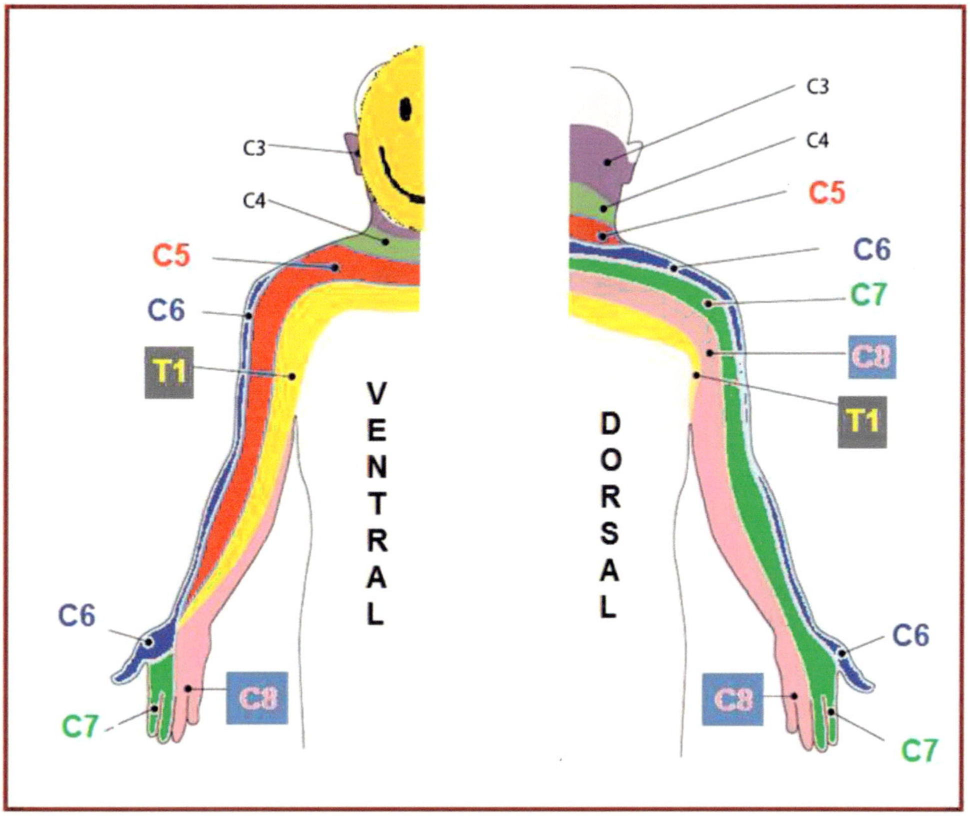

Figure 6: Dermatomes of the upper extremity. (Modified from http://www.cmej.org.za/index.php/cmej/article/view/2708/2829)

There may also be weakness and abnormal reflexes, as follows:

- C5: Deltoid and biceps weakness. Decreased biceps reflex.
- C6: Brachioradialis and wrist extension weakness. Decreased brachioradialis reflex.
- C7: Triceps and wrist flexion weakness. Decreased triceps reflex.
- C8: Intrinsic hand muscle weakness.

OBJECTIVE EVIDENCE

In evaluating patients for cervical stenosis, myelopathy or radiculopathy, radiographic images are crucial, starting with a cervical x-ray series (lateral, AP, oblique, and flexion/extension views are commonly used). Cervical stenosis can be categorized as "absolute stenosis" when the spinal canal diameter measures less than 10mm, or as "relative stenosis" when the diameter is 10 to 13mm. Stenosis is also suggested with a Torg-Pavlov ratio <0.8.

Cervical x-rays (Figure 7) may show significant degenerative changes such as osteophytes, disc space narrowing or facet joint hypertrophy.

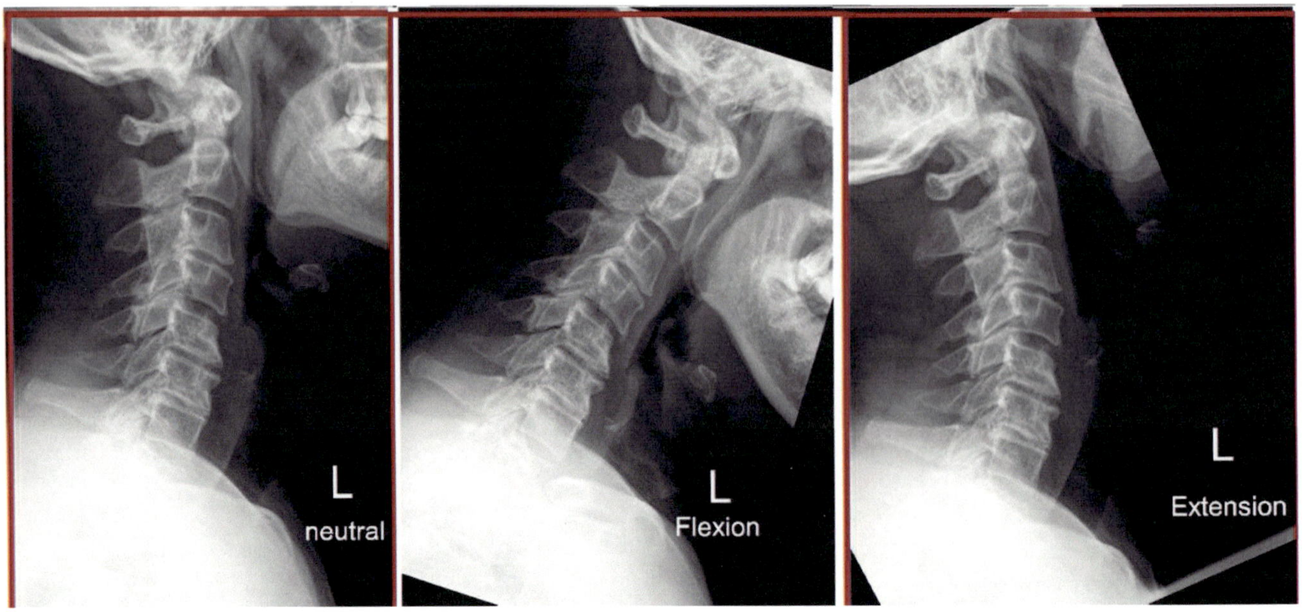

Figure 7: lateral radiograph showing spondylosis (degenerative disc space narrowing and osteophytic spurring) in the cervical spine. On flexion, there is an anterolisthesis of C4 with respect to C5 secondary to degenerative facet joints; this likely contributes to canal stenosis at C4/5. (Case and caption courtesy of Dr Yi-Jin Kuok, Radiopaedia.org, rID: 18348)

CT without contrast can provide information on the cervical vertebrae and cervical stenosis, but the limited soft tissue information reduces its utility. CT myelography can be used to visualize the space around the neural elements in patients with contraindications to MRI. In this test, a contrast medium is injected into the intradural space. Because this is an invasive test, it should be employed with proper prudence.

MRI is the study of choice for evaluating spinal cord or root compression (Figure 8). However, false positive findings are common. (Note that many asymptomatic people greater than 40 years of age will have some MRI abnormality). Findings must be evaluated in the context of appropriate presentation, and thus MRI should not be used as a screening test but to answer a specific clinical question.

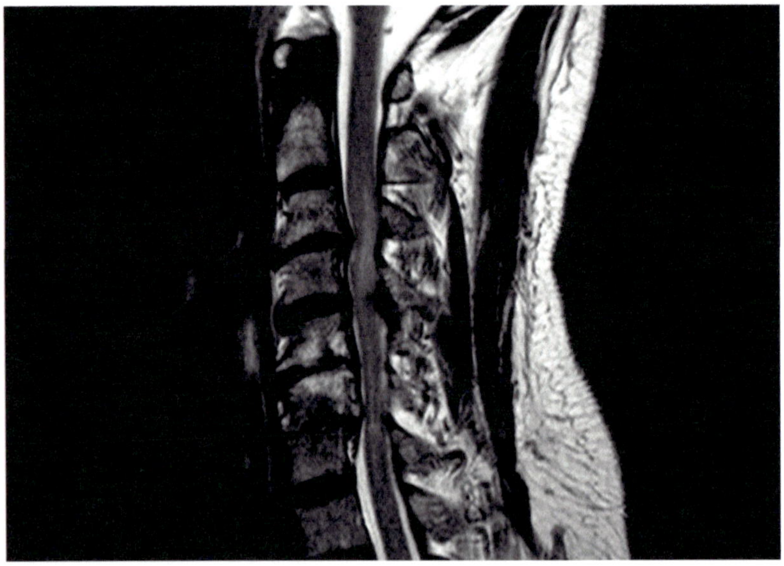

Figure 8: MRI showing cervical canal stenosis worse at C3/4 due to posterior osteophyte disc complex. There is associated spinal cord edema corresponding to myelopathy. (Case courtesy of Dr Yi-Jin Kuok, Radiopaedia.org, rID: 18348)

Electromyogram and nerve conduction studies can be used to localize peripheral nerve damage, however these studies are often operator-dependent and is unpleasant for many patients. This test should be used only to answer a specific question about treatment, and certainly not to rule-out cervical pathology. EMG/

NCV is useful when trying to determine the extent of peripheral nerve involvement in patients with cervical myelopathy.

No specific lab findings exist for myelopathy or radiculopathy.

EPIDEMIOLOGY

Cervical spine stenosis, though often asymptomatic, is quite common in the general population and correlates with age, as degenerative changes of aging (spondylosis) is the most common cause of stenosis. An estimated 5% of the general adult population, 7% of those over 50 years of age, and 9% of those over 70 years of age have cervical stenosis.

The exact proportion of people with asymptomatic cord compression that will go on to develop symptoms is not known. A prospective study of 199 people with cord compression seen on an MRI obtained because of neck pain or radiculopathy yet who did not show signs of myelopathy found that about 25% developed myelopathy within 2 years.

Because degenerative change is often the cause of cervical myelopathy, this condition has an increasing prevalence with age. Both sexes are affected equally by cervical myelopathy, although males usually have earlier onset of symptoms (50s in men vs 60s in women). Myelopathy is responsible for approximately 4 hospitalizations per 100,000 people per year in the US.

The prevalence of cervical radiculopathy also increases with age. The incidence rate peaks between 50 to 59 years of age. Overall, the annual incidence is approximately 85 cases per 100,000 people per year in the US, with a 2:1 male to female incidence ratio.

DIFFERENTIAL DIAGNOSIS

When myelopathy and/or radiculopathy are suspected, the following should be considered:

- Movement disorders: more common in the elderly. Symptoms such as tremors or, bradykinesia are clues.
- Vitamin B12 deficiency can present with numbness, tingling, and decreased proprioception. However, motor symptoms are usually absent or mild.
- Multiple sclerosis: can present with weakness and sensory abnormalities that are non-dermatomal. However, symptoms are most often remitting-relapsing rather than progressive as myelopathy and radiculopathy are.
- A stroke affecting the motor and/or sensory cortex may present similarly to myelopathy or radiculopathy. However, neck pain is not a component of strokes and other neurologic deteriorations (changes in mental status, aphasia, etc.) are likely to be present in cases of stroke.
- Peripheral nerve syndromes: Carpal tunnel syndrome (median nerve), Cubital tunnel syndrome (ulnar nerve), and other peripheral nerve compression/injury syndromes may present with dermatomal, unilateral symptoms that may be confused with radiculopathy. If physical exam findings are ambiguous, an EMG with NCS may help localize the area of nerve damage.

RED FLAGS

- Any weakness or sensory symptoms after trauma to the neck. Make sure to obtain imaging to rule out fractures or instability.
- History of cancer. There may be metastasis to the cervical spine or brain.
- Neurological deficits beyond just extremity weakness or numbness. Must evaluate for stroke or other

vascular pathologies.

TREATMENT OPTIONS AND OUTCOMES

The presence of asymptomatic cervical stenosis detected incidentally on imaging is not an indication for treatment.

Patients with mild disease with little-to-no functional impairment or moderate disease with contraindications for surgery can be treated with rest, NSAIDs and muscle relaxant medication. If there is weakness, physical therapy of the neck and affected extremities are beneficial.

Patients with radiculopathy may benefit from selective nerve root corticosteroid injections.

When patients' symptoms are severe or function markedly impaired, operative measures should be considered. The basic goal of all operative interventions is decompression of the spinal cord or the nerve root(s) and thereby preventing progression and restoring function. Multiple surgical techniques exist, including anterior decompression and fusion (Figure 9); laminectomy with posterior fusion; laminoplasty, in which a portion of the lamina is removed to enlarge the neural foramina; and prosthetic disc replacement (Figure 10).

Anterior cervical discectomy and fusion is indicated for persistent radicular pain that has not resolved with conservative management. This surgery is highly successful for single level disease, but with substantial multilevel disease, the surgery is more likely to fail. (The name of the operation is "fusion," but is more accurately be termed "attempted fusion:" especially with surgery at multiple levels, not always do the bones unite as hoped.)

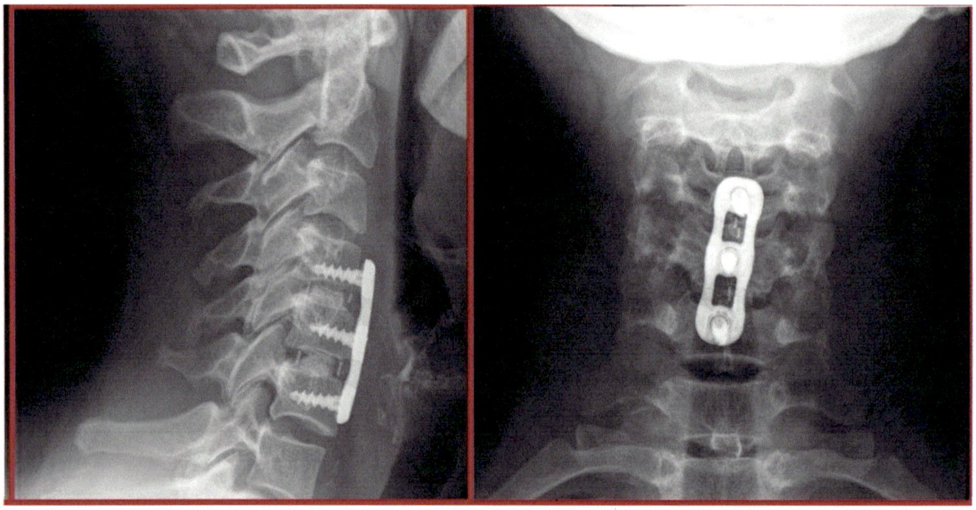

Figure 9: AP (right) and lateral (left) radiographs showing a plate and screws holding a cervical anterior cervical discectomy and fusion. (Case courtesy of Assoc Prof Craig Hacking, Radiopaedia.org, rID: 38120)

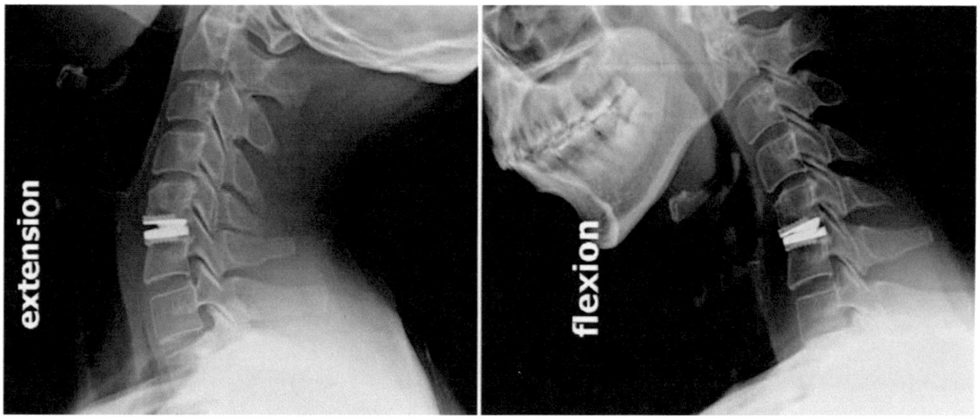

Figure 10: Extension and flexion radiographs showing an artificial disc with preserved segmental motion. (From https://bmcmusculoskeletdisord.biomedcentral.com/articles/10.1186/s12891-019-2509-0)

Non-operative treatment produces good outcomes in patients with mild symptoms as well as in those with larger spinal cord areas (>70mm2). Up to 75% of patients with radiculopathy will recover with just non-operative measures, as the herniated disc and associated compression/inflammation of the nerve roots may resolve over time. However, in patients with severe symptoms, non-operative treatments usually fail.

The majority of patients with radiculopathy resolve their symptoms after operative intervention (more than 90% in some studies). Many patients with myelopathy also report improvements in overall pain and symptoms with operative treatment, but the success rate is lower.

Procedures involving a fusion of three or more vertebral bodies place the cervical levels above and below the fusion at risk for accelerated degeneration. This is termed "adjacent segment disease."

Holistic Medicine

A report from the Mayo Clinic (https://www.mayoclinic.org/tests-procedures/chiropractic-adjustment/about/pac-20393513, visited 7/15/2021), suggests that chiropractic adjustments might be ill-advised for cervical spondylosis. This report claimed that "Serious complications associated with chiropractic adjustment are overall rare, but may include ...a herniated disk or a worsening of an existing disk herniation...[and] a certain type of stroke after neck manipulation." Patients were therefore advised to not seek chiropractic adjustment if they have "numbness, tingling, or loss of strength in an arm or leg" or "a known bone abnormality in the upper neck."

RISK FACTORS AND PREVENTION

The most common risk factor for cervical myelopathy and radiculopathy are age-related degenerative changes. Cervical canal stenosis, whether primary or secondary, is also an independent risk factor for developing myelopathy.

Smoking is the main modifiable risk factor for radiculopathy.

Reducing stress on the cervical spine through maintaining good posture and avoiding excessive loading can theoretically help slow the progression of the degeneration, although this is unproven.

MISCELLANY

The "Double crush hypothesis" maintains that compression of a nerve root in the cervical spine may make the distal nerve it supplies more susceptible to impairment. In particular, in the presence of cervical spondylosis or a cervical disc herniation, a patient may develop carpal tunnel syndrome from a lesser degree of median nerve compression than is ordinarily needed. The thought is that the proximal compression disrupts axonal transport along the nerve. This is intuitively appealing, but not proven. (It is likely that the hypothesis will remain unproved: proving causality would require sham-controlled, experimentally-induced nerve root compression, and that would be ethically impermissible.)

KEY TERMS

Spondylosis, myelopathy, radiculopathy, dermatome

SKILLS

Perform a comprehensive neurologic exam, including a detailed sensory exam, to determine whether symptoms are dermatomal or non-dermatomal in nature. Know the dermatome map of the cervical nerve roots. Be familiar with provocative physical exam maneuvers that may help distinguish cervical spine pathologies from isolated shoulder/arm pathologies.

CHAPTER 5.

EARLY ONSET SCOLIOSIS

Scoliosis is defined as a three-dimensional deformity of the spine that includes not only a more noticeable lateral deviation, but also rotation of the vertebrae within the (lateral) curvature. Scoliosis can be further classified by the age of a patient. Early onset scoliosis is defined as scoliosis diagnosed before the age of 10 years old due to any cause (Figure 1). Early onset scoliosis can be categorized by etiology: namely, congenital, syndromic, neuromuscular and idiopathic. The scoliosis might be present without a known cause too; this is termed idiopathic scoliosis. Idiopathic scoliosis is rare in children under the age of 10. (Adolescent idiopathic scoliosis is discussed in its own chapter.)

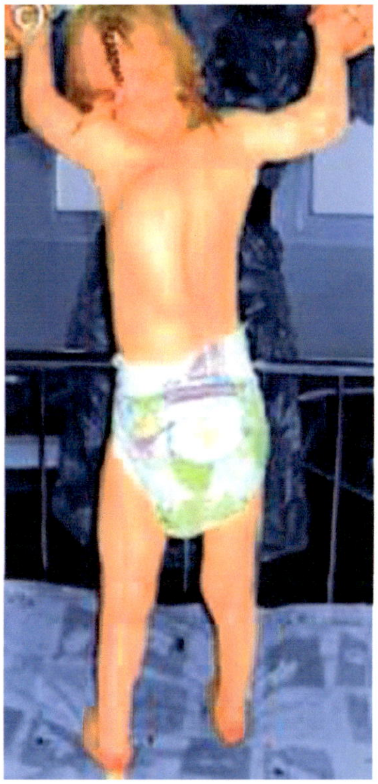

Figure 1. Clinical photograph of a two-year-old girl with severe thoracic early-onset scoliosis (Courtesy of Treatment strategies for early-onset scoliosis. EFORT Open Reviews. 3. 287-293. 10.1302/2058-5241.3.170051.)

STRUCTURE AND FUNCTION

Growth of the spine and the chest wall are critical for lung growth and development. Without normal growth, alveolar hypoplasia and disturbance of chest wall function causes a restrictive lung disease and possible respiratory failure.

The "golden time" for lung growth is from birth to the age of 5 years old and coincides with the period of most rapid growth of the thoracic spine and rib cage. Bronchial tree and alveolar complement are maximally developed by 8 years of age, and the thoracic volume at 10 years of age is 50% of the expected adult volume.

Patients with congenital anomalies causing their early onset scoliosis often have rib fusions or other anomalies that can disturb the normal biomechanics of chest wall, leading to decreased forced vital capacity (FVC). The term *thoracic insufficiency syndrome* (TIS) has been coined to describe the inability of the thorax to support normal respiration and lung growth.

Because the earlier that a spinal deformity appears, the greater the disturbance on thoracic cage, patients with early onset scoliosis have greater lung dysfunction and increased mortality rates compared to the general population, in proportion to the magnitude of the spinal deformity.

Early onset scoliosis can be categorized by etiology, as follows: congenital, syndromic, neuromuscular and idiopathic.

Congenital early onset scoliosis

Congenital scoliosis (Figure 2) is defined as scoliosis caused by at least one bony anomaly of the spine which is present at birth (though the diagnosis may not be made until later in childhood). Congenital anomalies include failure of vertebral formation, such as hemivertebrae or wedged vertebrae, or failure of separation or segmentation, such as block vertebrae or unilateral bars. A unilateral unsegmented bar with a contralateral hemivertebrae is the anomaly known for the worst risk of progression of congenital scoliosis. A positive family history is found in 1% of patients with congenital spinal deformities, but a genetic cause has not been discovered.

The neural axis, vertebral column, and other organ systems develop simultaneously at about five to eight weeks of gestation. Thus, congenital scoliosis may be associated with an intraspinal anomaly such as a tethered cord, diastematomyelia (a longitudinal cleft in the spinal cord), diplomyelia (duplication of the spinal cord), syringomyelia (fluid-filled cavity in the spinal cord), or Arnold-Chiari malformation (herniated cerebellar tonsils at the foramen magnum). Because the vertebral malformations form during embryogenesis at the same time the heart and kidneys are also developing, about 60% of patients will have abnormalities affecting these systems. Accordingly, a renal ultrasound and echocardiogram is often obtained to evaluate for concomitant pathology.

A constellation of symptoms often diagnosed in patients with congenital scoliosis is the VACTERL syndrome, consisting of: vertebral defects, anal atresia, cardiac defects, tracheo-esophageal fistula, renal anomalies, and limb abnormalities. A patient must have at least three of the features to be diagnosed with VACTERL syndrome.

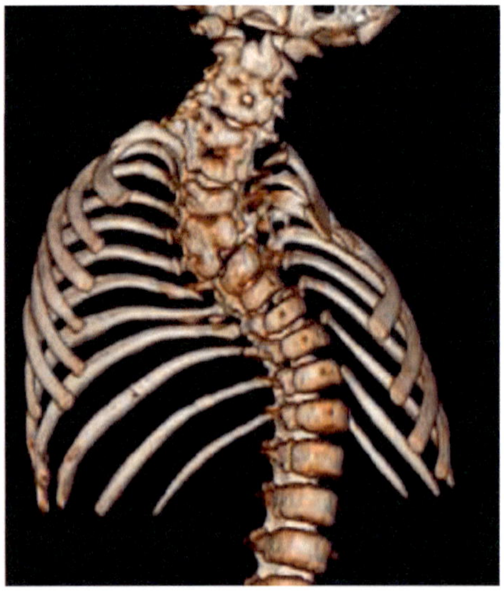

Figure 2: A 3-dimensional reconstruction of a CT scan demonstrating congenital scoliosis with fused ribs. (Courtesy of Treatment strategies for early-onset scoliosis. EFORT Open Reviews. 3. 287-293. 10.1302/2058-5241.3.170051.)

Syndromic early onset scoliosis

Syndromic scoliosis is defined as scoliosis that appears in conjunction with a recognized pediatric syndrome, such as Marfan's, Ehlers-Danlos, trisomy 21 (Downs syndrome), Prader-Willi, Retts, neurofibromatosis, Noonan, or osteoporosis imperfecta.

When a child is diagnosed with a syndrome known to be associated with scoliosis, it is important that physicians screen for scoliosis. The natural history of scoliosis associated with these syndromes varies, so the curves they cause progress at different rates and require personalized treatment approaches.

Neuromuscular early onset scoliosis

Neuromuscular scoliosis is defined as scoliosis caused by a neurologic disorder of the central nervous system or muscle, such as muscular dystrophy, cerebral palsy, spina bifida, spinal muscular atrophy, or Freidrich's ataxia.

The likelihood of developing neuromuscular scoliosis usually depends on the extent of nerve and muscle involvement with a specific disorder. Not all children with a neuromuscular disorder will develop scoliosis, but it is especially common in those who are not able to walk.

Neuromuscular scoliosis differs in particular from other types of scoliosis as the deformity is often a long, sweeping curve, typically involving the thoracic spine, the lumbar spine, as well as the pelvis.

Idiopathic early onset scoliosis

Idiopathic scoliosis is defined as scoliosis without known cause; that is, when congenital, syndromic and neuromuscular causes have been excluded. Children with idiopathic early onset scoliosis are considered otherwise healthy.

Idiopathic scoliosis can be of the infantile type (diagnosed at less than 3 years of age). This is very rare. Juvenile Idiopathic scoliosis is that diagnosed between 3 years and 10 years of age. (The most common form of idiopathic scoliosis, the Adolescent type, refers to scoliosis occurring after 10 years of age in the setting of an otherwise healthy child. This, by definition, is not a type of early onset scoliosis.)

PATIENT PRESENTATION

Evaluation of a patient with concern for early onset scoliosis begins with a comprehensive prenatal and birth history, as well as a detailed review of other medical conditions.

It is important that neurologic, pulmonary, urogenital, cardiovascular, and gastrointestinal systems have been evaluated if there is concern for congenital scoliosis.

If surgery is ultimately planned, evaluation should also include the current nutritional and pulmonary status of the patient.

A physical exam should start with measurements of height and weight. A full neurologic exam tests sensation, motor function and reflexes in the upper and lower extremities. Increased or decreased tone should be noted in patients with neuromuscular conditions. The skin should be examined for cafe-au-lait spots associated with neurofibromatosis, hair tufts or skin dimples near the sacrum associated with congenital scoliosis, and hypermobility associated with connective tissue disorders.

Coronal and sagittal balance is assessed by observing the patient from the front and the side, to see if they are tilted to one side (coronal imbalance), or have increased or decreased lordosis or kyphosis (sagittal imbalance). The examiner should also assess whether the torso is level, by palpating the iliac crests and the top of the shoulders.

The Adams forward bend test (Figure 3) has the patient bend at the waist, reaching toward their toes while the examiner stands behind the patient, looking at the back for asymmetric axial rotation of the trunk. If present, this will appear as a rib prominence on one side of the back. When the patient bends forward with the shoulders level with the hips, a scoliometer –a device similar to a carpenter's level, with a cutout to rest on the spine and markings to indicate the angular deviation from the horizontal– is laid to rest atop the most severe part of the deformity. A scoliometer reading of seven degrees or more warrants a referral to a pediatric orthopaedist.

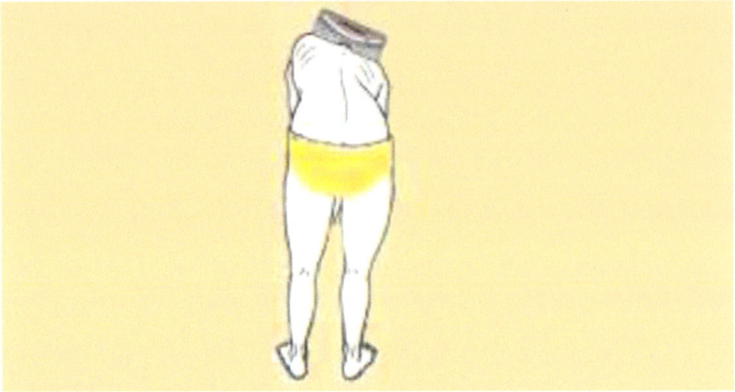

Figure 3: The Adams forward bending test, showing a scoliometer resting on the child's back as she bends forward. As shown, the scoliometer is approximately 20 degrees off the horizontal, a clearly abnormal value. (Modified under a Creative Commons Attribution 4.0 International License from Application of two-parameter scoliometer values for predicting scoliotic Cobb angle. BioMed Eng OnLine 16, 136 (2017). https://doi.org/10.1186/s12938-017-0427-7)

Note that performing the Adams forward bend test can be challenging in many children with EOS that are not independently ambulating; others may be unable to stay still for the scoliometer readings. In these cases, the spine exam can be performed while the child is sitting, with the examiner paying particular attention to shoulder or waistline asymmetry

OBJECTIVE EVIDENCE

The diagnosis of scoliosis is established with a plain radiograph in the posteroanterior plane. A lateral radiograph is also useful for evaluating for sagittal plane abnormalities and where a diagnosis of scoliosis is suspected. These two views should be obtained in most cases.

Radiographs are important to the diagnosis of congenital scoliosis because bony anomalies can be identified that are causing scoliosis to occur. In the absence of congenital anomalies, plain radiographs are useful for assessing the severity of scoliosis and the risk of progression.

The Cobb angle (Figure 4) describes the angle of the spinal curvature for each curve present in the spinal column resulting in a scoliosis. A patient may have cervicothoracic, thoracic, thoracolumbar, or lumbar curve(s) depending on which region of the spine is involved in scoliosis.

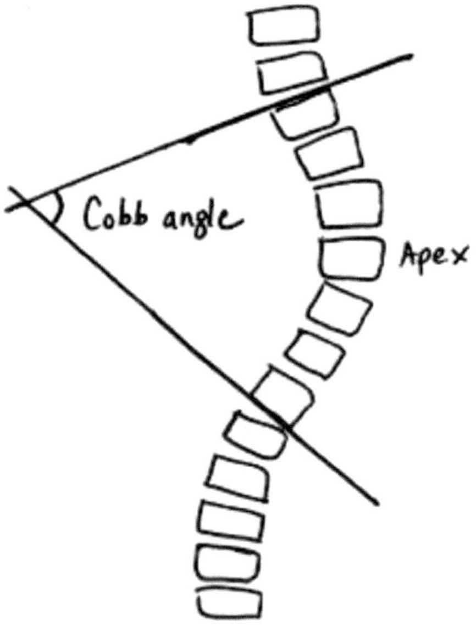

Figure 4: The Cobb angle, as shown, quantifies the magnitude of the curve.

To measure the Cobb angle, one must first decide which vertebrae are the end vertebrae of the curve deformity, which means the vertebra whose endplates are most tilted towards each other. Lines are then drawn along the endplates, and the angle between where the two lines intersect is the Cobb angle.

The vertebrae are also evaluated for the presence or absence of rib head overlap with the vertebral body at the apex of the curve (the vertebra that is located at the farthest point laterally from the midline of the body on the convexity of the curve). This assessment is termed the rib phase (Figure 5).

Phase 1 ribs do not overlap the vertebral bodies, while Phase 2 ribs do overlap the vertebral bodies. Patients with Phase 2 ribs are more likely to have progressive scoliosis, and therefore should be treated more aggressively.

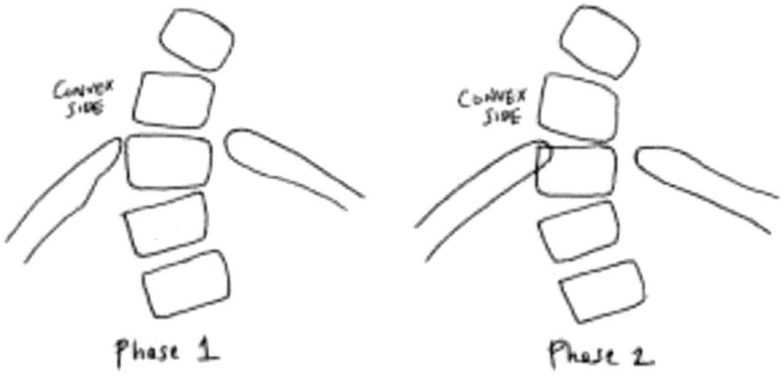

Figure 5: Phase 1 ribs, as shown to the left, do not overlap the vertebral bodies, whereas Phase 2 ribs, at right, do overlap the vertebral bodies.

An MRI of the entire spine is indicated for all patients with early onset scoliosis to evaluate for intraspinal abnormalities that may not yet be detectable based on clinical exam. About 20-40% of early onset scoliosis patients will have an abnormality, such as a tethered cord, Chiari malformation, or syrinx. A CT, especially with a three-dimensional reconstruction, can be useful to better delineate bony abnormalities and for surgical planning.

EPIDEMIOLOGY

More than 100,000 children in the United States are diagnosed with scoliosis annually. The majority of those children are diagnosed with adolescent idiopathic scoliosis rather than early onset scoliosis. Because early onset scoliosis comprises a group of conditions with diverse etiologies and natural histories, the exact prevalence of early onset scoliosis is unknown. Idiopathic early onset scoliosis is estimated to account for less than one percent of all scoliosis.

RED FLAGS

There are several "red flags" in the history, physical exam, and radiographs of a patient that should concern the treating provider.

An abnormal neurologic finding or a left thoracic curve can be predictive of an underlying pathologic condition of the spinal cord, although in early onset scoliosis, left thoracic curves are more common and less likely to be pathologic than in AIS.

A painful scoliosis should prompt suspicion for an osteoid osteoma, a benign bone tumor that in the spine is most commonly found in the thoracic and lumbar posterior elements and releases prostaglandin.

A rapidly-progressing scoliosis should raise concern for a tethered cord, also known as "tethered spinal cord syndrome." A tethered cord syndrome is present when there is a pathological development of excess fibrous connective tissue (fibrosis) in the filum terminale that fixes (or tethers) on the caudal spinal cord to the sacrum, limiting its movement. When a child grows, this abnormal attachment causes stretching and tension on the spinal cord. This can cause scoliosis, motor and sensory changes in the legs, back pain, foot deformities, and urinary dysfunction. Scoliosis can be one of the early signs of a tethered cord, so if there is any concern then an MRI should be ordered.

TREATMENT OPTIONS AND OUTCOMES

Historically, the standard of care for severe, progressive early onset scoliosis was early definitive anterior and posterior spinal instrumented fusion. It was thought that a short but straight spine was superior to a long but curved spine, but now our understanding is that a well-aligned spine with a thoracic cavity large enough to support pulmonary development is the proper goal.

Nutrition is important in early onset scoliosis patients independent of treatment. Patients with severe spine deformity are often underweight, have poor soft tissue coverage over rib or spinal bony prominences/implants, and thus are a setup for complications. A nutrition consult can be helpful in advance of any treatment or at the time of the occurrence of wound complications in order to best optimize the patient pre-operatively or promote healing moving forward.

Non-operative Treatment

The first approach to a patient with early onset scoliosis is to use non-operative methods in an attempt to delay surgery. Some patients will in fact improve with non-operative treatment alone, such that later surgery is not needed. About 80% of children with idiopathic infantile scoliosis, for instance, will have resolution of scoliosis.

Serial casting and bracing have both been used. The concept of serial casting is based on the fact that growth can drive correction of the three-dimensional deformity. Patients with documented progression of scoliosis but low magnitude curvature (less than 60 degrees) or low risk for anticipated progression are candidates for serial casting.

A cast is applied on a special table that applies traction to the patient's head and legs while anesthetized. The traction distracts the facet joints so that there can be increased movement between vertebrae, then the cast is applied with a mold over the ribs in order to rotate the spine and chest wall opposite the direction of the deformity. Windows are made in the cast anteriorly and posteriorly to allow room for normal expansion of the thoracic and abdominal cavities with respiration and eating. Casts are changed every 2 to 4 months based on age and growth and can be eventually replaced by a brace if the curve reduces to 10 to 20 degrees.

Outcomes of casting are best when casting is initiated at a younger age and when performed for less severe, idiopathic curves. Concerns and potential complications of casting include skin breakdown, negative effects on quality of life, repetitive anesthesia events for cast changes, and superior mesenteric artery or brachial plexus compression from the cast. Casts may not be tolerated in patients with poor pulmonary function or sensory disorders. Bracing can be similarly used to control non-congenital early onset scoliosis deformities with a goal of delaying surgery, or after serial casting is successfully completed. When a brace is used in a rapidly growing child younger than 5 years old, the patient may develop rib deformity or loss of the normal sagittal profile from pressure from the brace.

Operative Treatment

Currently, the concept of allowing continued growth of the spine and chest instead of performing a spinal fusion, while still managing spinal deformity, is of great interest in early onset scoliosis patients. Growth-sparing techniques have been classified into distraction-based techniques (meaning distracting posteriorly on the spine to lengthen the spine and enlarge the thoracic cavity), convex compression-based growth inhibition (meaning inhibiting vertebral body growth on the convexity of the curve to correct a curve), and guided growth (meaning directing growth to correct a curve over time). Spinal fusion is typically delayed until at least age 10, at which point the thoracic cavity is sufficiently developed to support the child through adult life.

Distraction-based techniques involve attaching rods to the spine or ribs proximally and to the spine or pelvis distally, while avoiding the spine in between the anchored segments. The rods are then distracted or lengthened by various mechanisms in order to produce growth of the spine and in turn the thoracic cavity. The options for distraction-based instrumentation include the "vertical expandable prosthetic titanium rib," also known as the VEPTR, (Figure 6); a "traditional growing rod" (TGR) (Figure 7); and the magnetically-controlled growing rod (MCGR) (Figure 8).

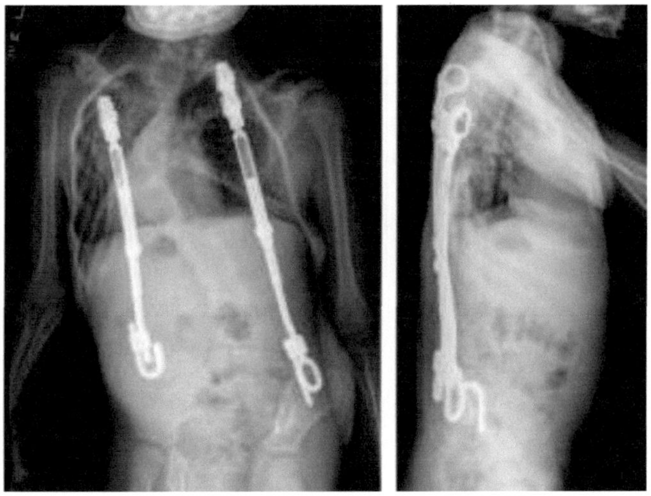

Figure 6: A patient with bilateral vertical expandable prosthetic titanium rib devices, VEPTRs, placed for congenital scoliosis and thoracic insufficiency syndrome. The VEPTR is a rib-distraction device that was designed specifically to address the thoracic insufficiency by expanding the thoracic cavity. As the child grows, VEPTR adjustment (under anesthesia) is performed every 6-8 months until the child reaches skeletal maturity.

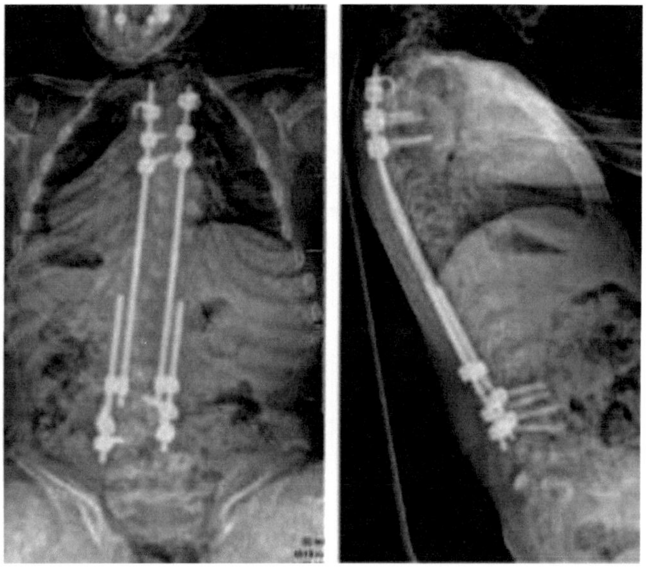

Figure 7: A patient with bilateral traditional growing rods. In the technique, a combination of hooks, wires and screws are anchored both proximally and distally to the spine via a short fusion and are connected by tunneled rods beneath the soft tissue. This technique must be distracted surgically under anesthesia as well.

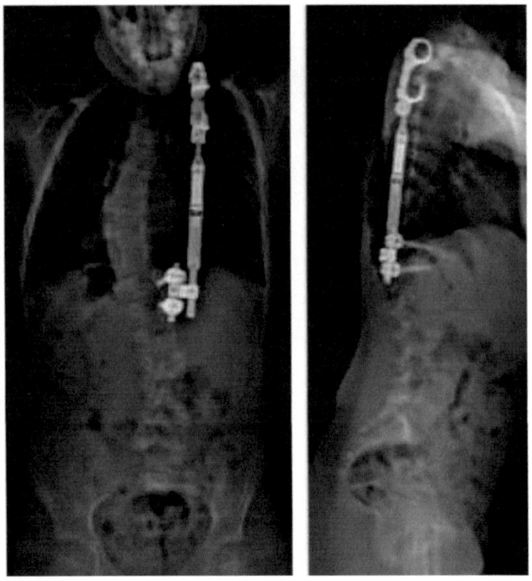

Figure 8: A patient with a unilateral magnetically-controlled growing rod, with rib anchors proximally and spine anchors distally. Magnetically-controlled growing rods are similar to traditional growing rods, with the notable difference being that the anchors can be distracted using a magnet in the out-patient setting.

Complications of these techniques include implant prominence which can eventually result in skin breakdown, surgical site infection, implant breakage, implant migration, and failure to lengthen, all of which result in return trips to the operating room and additional anesthetic events. Repeat lengthening surgery is problematic as with each additional surgical procedure the likelihood of a complication rises in an already risky/sick patient population. (This makes the MCGR so appealing: it helps avoid trips to the operating room.)

Convex compression-based growth inhibits deformity progression by applying a compressive force on the convex side of the scoliosis deformity.

Guided growth(Shilla system) relies on fixation at the apex of a scoliosis curve with gliding fixation proximally and distally so that the spine can continue to grow above and below while gradually correcting the scoliosis. Osteotomies are performed at the apex to correct as much deformity as possible and pedicle screws are placed at the apex over three or four vertebral segments.

Resection and short fusion can be the treatment methodology employed when attempting to manage specific types of congenital scoliosis. A hemivertebra causing a progressive scoliosis in a very young child may be completely resected with a short (2-level) spinal fusion using pedicle screws/hooks to correct deformity and minimize the need for repeat surgical procedures. However, there are risks of neurological injury with hemivertebra resection, thus the decision to resect versus growth-sparing techniques may be a complicated one.

KEY TERMS

Early onset scoliosis, congenital scoliosis, neuromuscular scoliosis, syndromic scoliosis, idiopathic scoliosis, casting, growth-sparing spine surgery

SKILLS

Name the etiologies of early onset scoliosis. Understand the importance of spinal growth on thoracic cavity growth and pulmonary development. Describe the Adams forward bend test and how to use a scoliometer. Describe VACTERL syndrome. Understand the work-up, associated conditions or syndromes, and red flags important for a patient with concern for early onset scoliosis. Understand the measurements used in radiographic assessment of early onset scoliosis and measure the Cobb angle in plain x-rays.

CHAPTER 6.

LUMBAR DISC DISEASE

The intervertebral discs in the lumbar spine may fail to remain within the borders defined by the vertebral bodies and in turn compress nerve roots. This process can be caused by trauma, degeneration or a combination of both. In laymen's terms, this condition is known as a 'slipped disc.' Disc pathology is a common cause of low back pain and radicular leg pain, typically affecting the L4-L5 and L5-S1 levels. Diagnosis is made by history and physical examination, with MRI confirmation. Non-operative management with NSAIDs and physical therapy is usually successful, though surgical decompression is indicated for disabling pain or progressive neurological deficits.

STRUCTURE AND FUNCTION

There are 23 spinal discs in the human body, found between adjacent vertebral bodies from C2 to S1. The discs absorb axial forces such as body weight and landing after jumping; they also aid in spinal movements such as flexing and twisting.

Intervertebral discs have a strong, fibrous outer layer, known as the annulus fibrosus, and a gel-like inner layer, known as the nucleus pulposus. Both the annulus fibrosus and the nucleus pulposus contain type-I collagen, proteoglycans and water. In the annulus fibrosus, there is more collagen relative to proteoglycan and water. The high collagen content gives the annulus fibrosus tensile strength. By contrast, the nucleus pulposus has more proteoglycan and water than collagen, and is accordingly particularly good at resisting compression and axial loads.

The normal disc lies wholly within the boundaries of the so-called disc space: this is defined above and below by the vertebral body end plates and peripherally by the outer edges of the vertebral body (see Figure 1).

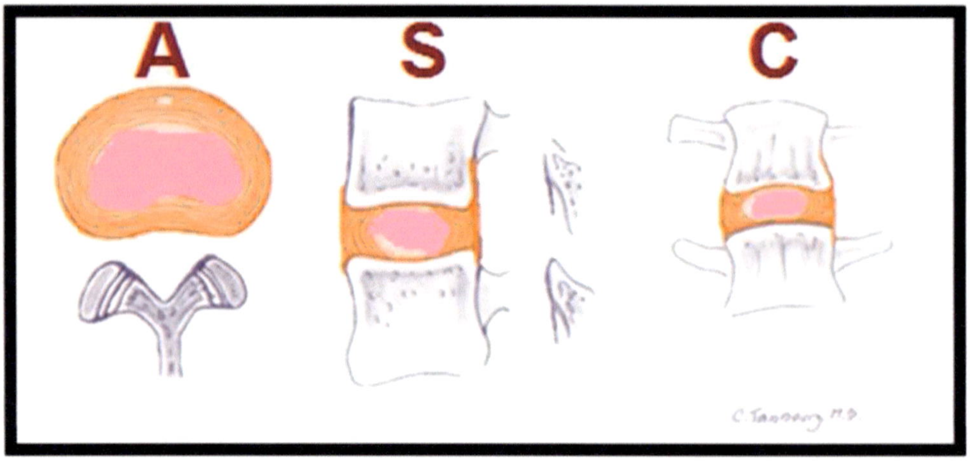

Figure 1: An axial (A), sagittal (S) and coronal (C) schematic view of the disc. The annulus fibrosus is shown in orange and the nucleus puposus in pink. As seen on the sagittal view (and implicit on the axial view as well), the posterior aspect of the disc is in line with the posterior aspect of the vertebral body. (Modified from Fardon; see acknowledgment below.)

According to the nomenclature recommended by the North American Spine Society, the American Society of Spine Radiology and the American Society of Neuroradiology, a disc that has left its disc space can be termed a "herniation" if there is focal displacement (representing < 25% of the disc circumference), or a "bulge" if the disc material is displaced throughout the circumference of the disc.

A disc herniation in turn can be classified as a *protrusion* or an *extrusion,* depending on the geometry of the disc material outside of the disc space. If the base is wider than the distance displaced, a protrusion is present, whereas with extrusion, the displaced disc is narrower than the base (see Figures 2 and 3).

Beyond that, extruded discs may lose their continuity with the disc from which they came. This is known as a *sequestered disc herniation.* Discs may also herniate into the vertebral body itself, via defects in the end plate. These are called intravertaebral herniations (see Figure 4).

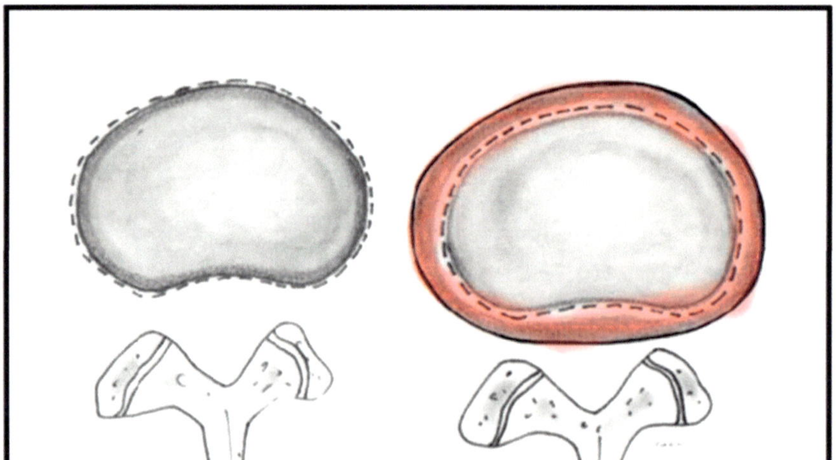

Figure 2: A bulging disc to the right, with a normal disc on the left. As shown in red, there is symmetric bulging of the annulus beyond the edges of the vertebral body, symmetrically throughout the circumference of the disc. (Modified from Fardon)

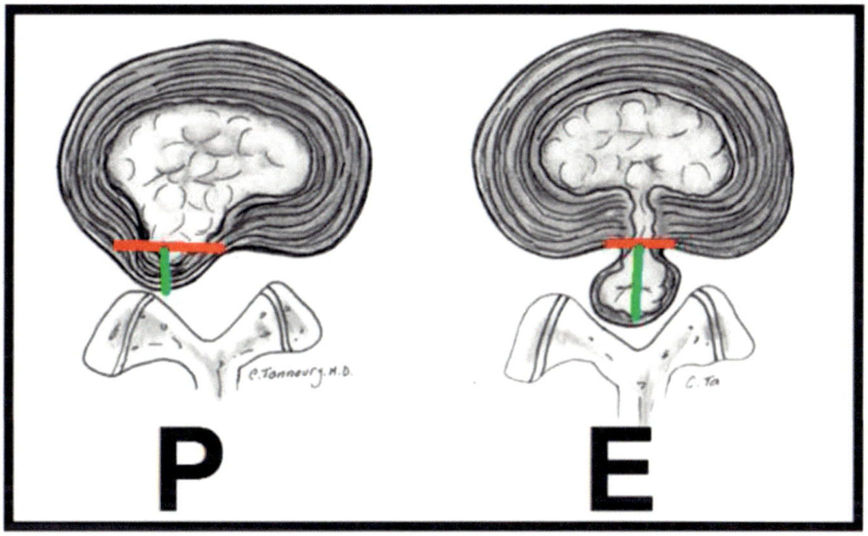

Figure 3: Axial views of a herniated disc: protrusion type (P) is shown at left, with an extrusion (E) shown in the right image. Contrasted with a bulge, with a herniation the disc displacement is focal. The distinction between protrusion and extrusion is that in the protrusion type the length of the displaced disc (green line) is less the width (red line). (Modified from Fardon.)

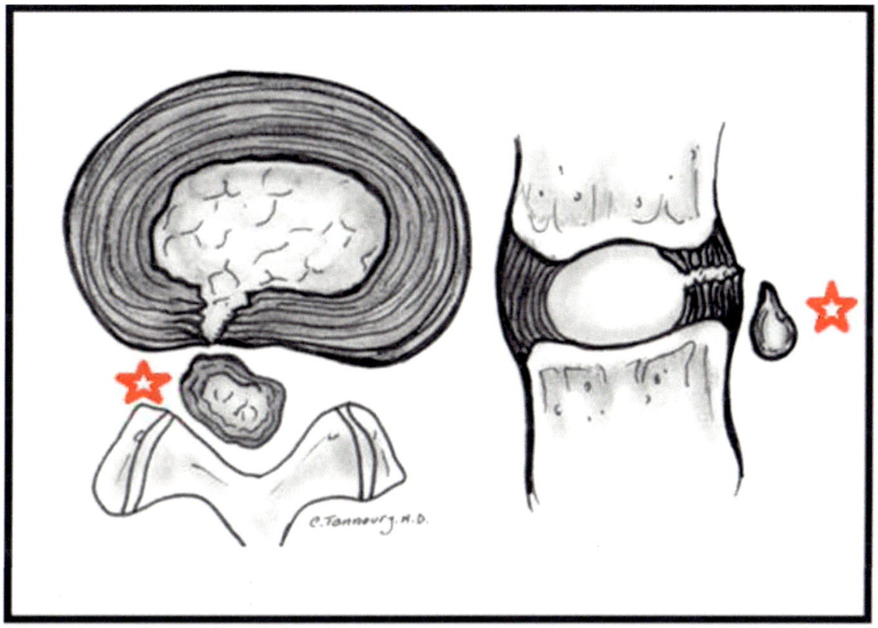

Figure 4: Axial (left) sagittal (right) images show a sequestered disc, cut off from the disc of origin (red star). (Modified from Fardon)Disc herniations occur when a tear in the annulus fibrosus allows the nucleus pulposus to push through this outer layer. The herniated material may compress the central spinal canal or nearby nerve roots. Herniations are most commonly posterolateral or paracentral (~90%) because the posterior longitudinal ligament (PLL) is weakest laterally. (Far lateral herniations that can enter the neural foramen directly represent the remaining 10%.)

Flexion of the spine causes compression of the anterior disc, potentially distending the material against the tensed posterior. When the PLL tears along with the annulus fibrosus, the herniation is considered "not contained." When the PLL fibers are weakened but still preserved, the herniation is "contained."

In the lumbar spine, the nerve roots are named by the level of the pedicle under which they exit the spine. For example, the L5 nerve root exits under the L5 pedicle (see Figure 5). Note that the nerve roots branch off the cauda equina [see below] within the central canal one level above their exit point, and descend vertically within the canal before exiting through the foramen. The L5 nerve, again by example, branches off the cauda equina between the L4 and L5 vertebrae, and travels distally across the L5 vertebral body before exiting laterally under the pedicle of L5. As such, L5 is subject to compression at two distinct places: by a central disc herniation of the L4/L5 disc, and (more commonly) by a lateral disc herniation at L5/S1.

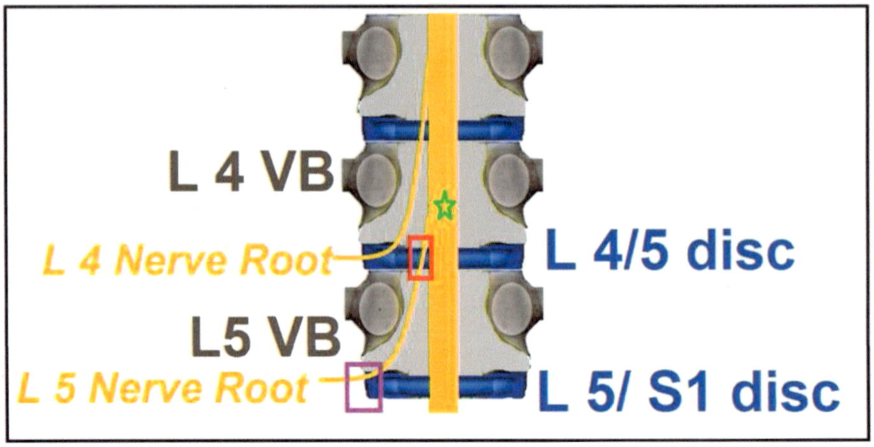

Figure 5: The lumbar nerve roots are shown. The branching off of the L5 root is shown by the green star, with the areas of central and lateral compression shown by the red and purple boxes, respectively.

(The lumbar arrangement lies in contrast to that of the cervical spine, where nerve roots transverse horizontally across one disc and exit under the pedicle of the body numbered *above* (so-called "mismatch"). That is, the C5 root exits under the C4 pedicle. Because of the root's horizontal path in the cervical spine, a herniation at C4-5 herniation will affect the C5 nerve root, if any, independent of whether the disc herniation is central or lateral).

Severe compression of the central spinal canal that causes severe stenosis is rare but can be a surgical emergency when the herniated material impinges on the cauda equina. Cases where the compression causes significant bilateral lower extremity motor/sensory deficits or bowel/bladder dysfunction requires urgent surgical intervention.

PATIENT PRESENTATION

Lumbar disc bulges and herniations can present as axial pain when associated with degenerative disc disease. If there is nerve root compression or irritation, patients might complain of pain or paresthesias traveling from the back to the buttock and down the posterior leg, so-called radicular symptoms. When the L4-L5 level is involved, pain may wrap around the leg to the dorsum of the foot. With L5-S1 herniations, symptoms are more commonly present on the plantar side of the foot. Muscle weakness may also be a complaint. Symptoms are usually unilateral but can be bilateral when large herniations are centrally located. Oftentimes, patients will describe worsening of pain with sitting or bending, a motion that exacerbates disc bulging.

The physical examination begins with an assessment of gait. Strength testing of the lower extremity muscles should be performed and graded on a 0 to 5 scale. Knee extension and ankle dorsiflexion tests L4 motor function, and physical exam for L4 nerve root injury may also reveal a weakened patellar reflex. L5 is the major nerve root controlling hip abduction and great toe extension (which may be easier to test). The S1 nerve root can be tested by having the patient toe walk: plantar flexion via gastrocnemius and soleus function relies on this nerve root.

Active and passive range of motion as well as strength testing of the hip can reveal abnormalities and is important to perform since hip pain is commonly mislabeled as back pain. Range of motion of the spine should be evaluated by flexion, extension, rotation, and bending to either side. Flexion of the spine increases the load on the posterior disc. This motion therefore usually results in worsening of pain or paresthesias when a disc herniation is present. In contrast, a worsening of symptoms on extension is more consistent with a diagnosis of degenerative arthritis. Tenderness to palpation over the paraspinal muscles and over the spinous processes is not specific for a herniated disc.

The straight leg raise is an important, albeit subjective, test for diagnosing L5 or S1 radiculopathy. With the patient lying supine, the examiner passively lifts the affected leg (straightened at the knee) from 30 to

70 degrees. If this maneuver reproduces the patient's radiating pain or paresthesias, it is considered positive. Pain reproduction when testing the contralateral leg (lifting the asymptomatic leg and causing pain of the symptomatic leg) has a higher specificity but lower sensitivity, so may be used for confirmation.

OBJECTIVE EVIDENCE

Disc herniation with radiculopathy can be diagnosed on clinical grounds, but is invariably diagnosed by MRI(Figure 6). MRI is both highly sensitive and specific for describing the anatomy, although it may detect findings that are clinically incidental. As such, MRI is best used to answer a specific clinical question, and not as a screening or surveillance modality.

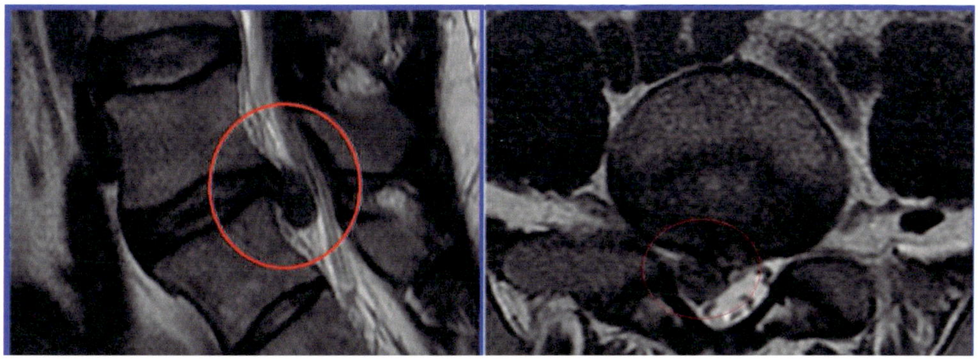

Figure 6: Sagittal (left) and axial (right) images of an extrude disc herniation [red circles]. (Case courtesy of Radiopaedia.org, rID: 2670)

MRI can help discern the cause of disc herniation. If there is imaging evidence of violent trauma and no evidence of degeneration, causality can be established. On the other hand, in the presence of degenerative changes and without significant imaging evidence of an associated violent injury such as fracture or dislocation, the Fardon task force (see *Acknoledgwments*, below) recommends classifying the disc herniation as degenerative rather than traumatic.

MRI with gadolinium should be obtained when considering revision surgery, because post-surgical scarring will enhance with contrast while recurrent disc herniation will not. Gadolinium is also necessary if there is suspicion of neoplastic or infectious etiology. If plain radiography is performed, findings may include narrowing of the space between adjacent vertebral bodies, loss of lumbar or cervical lordosis, or spondylosis.

Additionally, electrodiagnostic studies can help rule out peripheral neuropathy as the cause of extremity symptoms.

EPIDEMIOLOGY

More than 90% of disc herniations occur in the lumbar spine, due to its prominent role in flexion and extension. Most lumbar herniations are at the L4-L5 or L5-S1 levels. Lumbar disc herniations occur most frequently between the ages of 40 and 60, but can occur at almost any age after 18 years. Males have nearly a three times higher incidence of lumbar disc herniation.

Notably, many disc herniations may not cause symptoms. In the classic study of Boden et al [J Bone Joint Surg Am 1990 Mar;72(3):403-8.], about one-third of the population of asymptomatic volunteers were seen to have a "substantial abnormality" on MRI: of those who were less than sixty years old, 20% had a herniated disc and in the group that was sixty years old or older, 36% of the subjects had a disc herniation.

DIFFERENTIAL DIAGNOSIS

The differential diagnosis of disc herniation includes other causes of nerve root compression and inflammation, including spinal stenosis, mass lesions such as a tumor, fibrosis from previous surgery, and spondylolisthesis. Degenerative joint disease can produce bone spurs which may impinge on a nerve root. A hematoma should be considered in patients taking anticoagulants, who have recently had a spinal puncture procedure, or who have suffered trauma to the back.

Axial pain from facet joint degenerative joint disease usually presents as ill-defined pain, worse with activity and relieved with rest. Degenerative joint disease usually does not cause pain to radiate down the extremities, but some patients may describe low back pain traveling below the buttocks. Infectious etiologies such as osteomyelitis and discitis usually present as localized pain and do not radiate.

RED FLAGS

Cauda equina syndrome is a very rare and serious presentation of massive disc herniation in which the bundle of nerve roots at the end of the spinal cord are compressed within the spinal canal. The cauda equina consists of the nerve roots and rootlets that branch off of the lower end of the spinal cord (the conus medullaris). The cauda equina includes the nerve roots from lumbar and sacral regions. These nerve roots, although branched off the spinal cord itself at roughly the L1 vertebral level, remain within the central canal until they exit at their appropriate neural foramen. These nerves are said to resemble a horse's tail, hence the name cauda equina (Figure 7).

Cauda equina syndrome occurs when the nerves of the cauda equina are compressed by any space-occupying lesion, including a large herniated disc, tumor, epidural abscess, or bony protrusion. The compression of multiple nerves in the cauda equina often leads to unilateral or bilateral lower extremity pain and sensorimotor changes, bowel/bladder dysfunction, which can manifest as incontinence or urinary retention (with overflow incontinence and increased post-void residuals). Patients may also present with sexual dysfunction, saddle anesthesia, and absence of lower extremity reflexes.

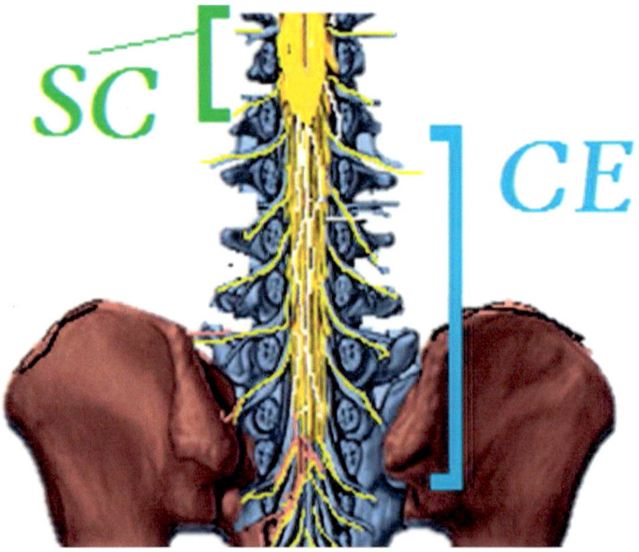

Figure 7: The cauda equina. The neural elements are shown in yellow. The region of the spinal cord (SC), ending usually at L1-L2, is identified by the green brackets, and that of the cauda equina (CE) distal to that.

Weight loss or a diagnosis of cancer elsewhere in the body are red flags for spinal metastases. A history of IV drug use, fevers, or an elevated WBC count should raise suspicion for an abscess, osteomyelitis, or discitis.

TREATMENT OPTIONS AND OUTCOMES

Nearly all patients will have sufficient improvement of symptoms within 3 months with non-operative care. Non-operative treatment includes the use NSAIDs or acetaminophen, exercise and dieting for weight loss, and physical therapy.

Patients should gradually increase activity as tolerated. Bedrest is unwise.

Second-line medications include muscle relaxants such as cyclobenzaprine or a corticosteroid taper.

Surgery should be reserved for patients who have failed non-operative therapy or patients with significant or progressive neurologic deficits, such as those with cauda equina syndrome.

Operative treatment includes hemilaminotomy and discectomy of which can be done in a traditional open manner or microsurgically. In traditional discectomy, a surgical incision is made that allows for removal of a portion of the lamina superficial to the herniated disc. The herniated material is then removed. A microdiscectomy is a similar procedure, but involves use of an operative microscope and special retractors for a smaller incision.

Post-operative rehabilitation is relatively simple, with the majority of patients returning to medium or high-intensity activity after 4 to 6 weeks. Complications of surgery include recurrent herniated disc (most common approximately 4% during the first year after surgery), dural tear (in 1-2% of patients), and discitis (less than 0.5% of patients).

The natural progression of a herniation is to decrease in size over time via reabsorption, which is mediated by macrophage phagocytosis. Within 3 months, over 90% of patients will see an improvement in their symptoms through non-operative treatment alone.

Laminotomy and discectomy have been shown to produce a significantly faster reduction in pain compared with non-operative treatment in observational studies. (Note that this result has not been shown in any sham trial, and thus a placebo effect might confound the result.) Factors associated with better surgical outcomes include a positive straight leg raise test pre-operatively, an MRI that is consistent with the patient's complaint of weakness, and leg pain as the primary symptom. Social factors may play a role too, as being married is also associated with better outcomes. When worker's compensation is involved in the case, surgical patients are less likely to see improvement in their symptoms and quality of life. Revision surgery outcomes for herniation recurrence are not significantly worse than primary surgery outcomes.

RISK FACTORS AND PREVENTION

The incidence of disc herniation increases with age. With aging, the vertebral discs lose water content and flexibility and the gel-like nucleus pulposus is replaced with fibrocartilage. Several genes have been implicated in the development accelerated degeneration including those coding for extracellular matrix proteins such as type I collagen, Vitamin D Receptor, and matrix metalloproteinases.

Obesity is associated with disc herniation due to the increased load placed on the spine. Likewise, a sedentary lifestyle, itself associated with obesity, is a risk factor for herniation as the seated position focuses pressure on the internal part of the disc.

Athletes playing contact sports are prone to disc herniation via sudden rotational movements and flexion of the spine.

Disease prevention is aimed at maintaining a healthy weight, strengthening core and back muscles for spine support, practicing good posture, and education on proper technique of lifting heavy objects (using one's legs and not bending over at the waist). Weightlifters should be encouraged to use support belts and to recognize signs of fatigue before they regress into improper lifting form.

MISCELLANY

Harrison Ford suffered a herniated disc while riding an elephant in Sri Lanka during the filming of *Indiana Jones: Temple of Doom.*

KEY TERMS

Herniated disc, annulus fibrosis, nucleus pulposus, radiculopathy, neck pain, low back pain, sciatica, straight leg raise, Spurling test, discectomy, cauda equina syndrome

SKILLS

Distinguish radicular pain from axial and referred low back pain by taking a focused history. Perform strength testing of ankle dorsiflexion, hallux extension, and ankle plantarflexion to distinguish between the L4, L5, and S1 level, respectively. Be able to perform a straight leg raise and contralateral straight leg raise to provoke lumbar radiculopathy. Know the red flags for low back pain and identify the indications for obtaining an MRI study.

Acknowledgement

This chapter draws heavily on the paper by Fardon et al, *Lumbar disc nomenclature: version 2.0: Recommendations of the combined task forces of the North American Spine Society, the American Society of Spine Radiology and the American Society of Neuroradiology*. Spine J. 2014 Nov 1;14(11):2525-45. https://pubmed.ncbi.nlm.nih.gov/24768732/

CHAPTER 7.

LUMBAR SPONDYLOSIS

Lumbar spondylosis, or degeneration of the lumbar discs and facet joints, is a common feature of aging. This degeneration often presents without causing symptoms beyond a routine back ache. However, the tissue overgrowth, ligamentum flavum hypertrophy, and bony osteophytes that accompany the degenerative process can also cause narrowing of the lumbar spinal canal (spinal stenosis). These processes can compress the neural elements causing leg pain, lower extremity numbness, buttock pain, and weakness.

Degeneration of the disc and facet capsule can also lead to instability and slippage of one vertebral body relative to the one below, a condition known as spondylolisthesis. This slippage can cause compression of the nerve roots in the canal as well, by narrowing the space occupied by the nerves.

STRUCTURE AND FUNCTION

The five lumbar vertebrae, designated L1 to L5, lie between the rib cage and the pelvis (see Figure 1). The central canal lies behind the body of each vertebra and is bordered by the pedicles and the laminae (see Figures 2 and 3). There is an intervertebral disc between the adjacent vertebra. There are also superior and inferior articular processes that make up the facet joint: the inferior articular process of the vertebrae above lying either dorsally (cervical and thoracic spine) or medially (lumbar spine) to the superior articular process of the vertebrae below.

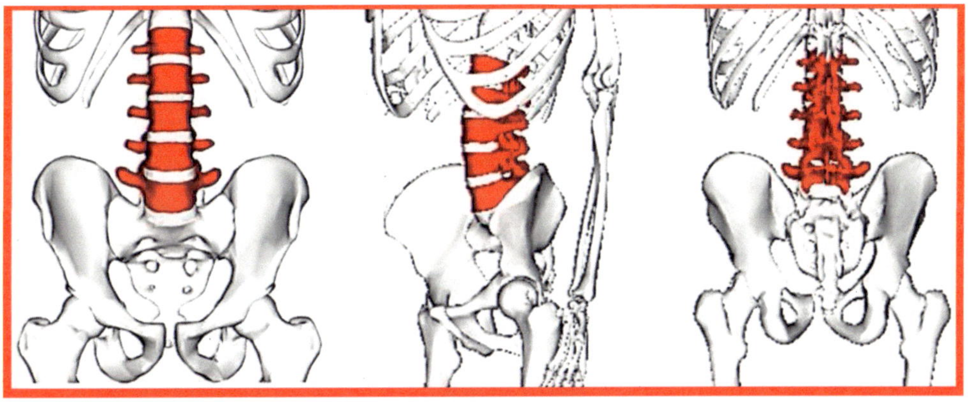

Figure 1: The lumbar spine, highlighted in red: anterior view (left) lateral oblique (center) and posterior view (right). (Courtesy of Wikipedia)

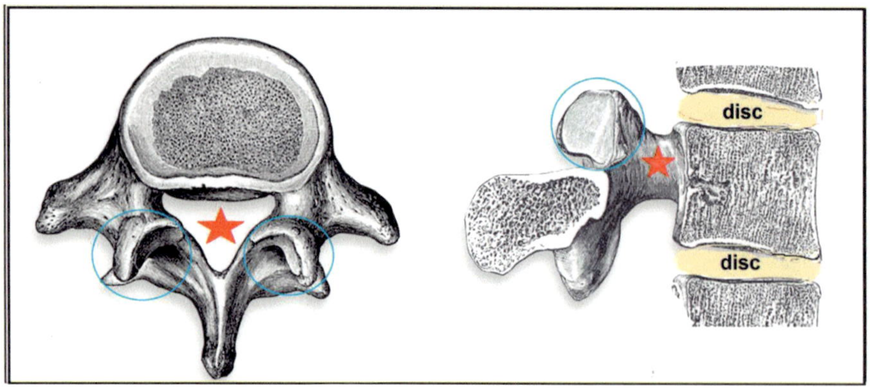

Figure 2: A lumbar vertebral body with superior view to the left and mid-sagittal view to the right. The central canal is denoted with a red star. The superior articular processes that make up the anterior side of the facet joints are circled in blue. The disc lies between the vertebral bodies, as shown. (Modified from Radiopaedia.org, rID: 82813/Gray's Anatomy)

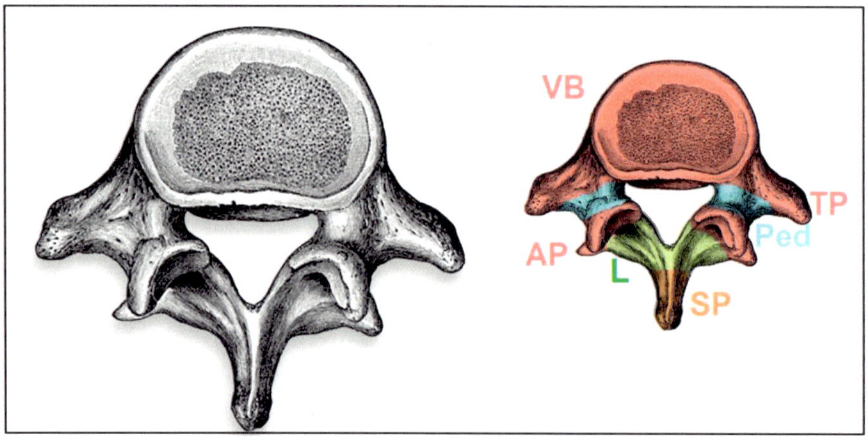

Figure 3: Colorized version of a superior view of a vertebra, highlighting the general area of the pedicles in blue, the laminae in green, and the spinous process in orange. The remaining bone, comprising the vertebral body, the articular processes, and transverse processes, are shown in red.

Along the vertebral column, there are anterior and posterior longitudinal ligaments adjacent to the vertebral bodies (see Figure 4). Posteriorly, the ligamentum flavum runs between adjacent lamina. Hypertrophy of the ligamentum flavum can compress the canal or the neural foramen and put pressure on the nerve roots.

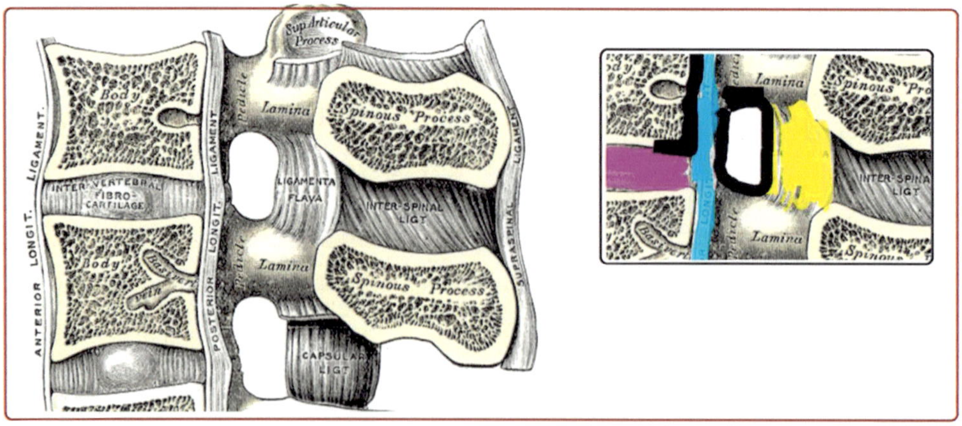

Figure 4: The ligaments of the lumbar spine. To the left is the original from Gray's Anatomy. To the right the potential sources of compression are shown in color: the disc in purple, the bony elements (see text) in black, the posterior longitudinal ligament in blue, and the ligamentum flavum (Latin for "yellow ligament") is shown (of course) in yellow.

Osteophytes (bone spurs) can form near the neural foramen as part of the degenerative process. These bone spurs may grow into the spinal canal resulting in central or lateral recess stenosis or grow into the foramen causing foraminal stenosis.

When the disc degenerates, it becomes flatter. This will shrink the size of the foramen inherently. As the disc space narrows, this will also alter the geometry of the facet joints. This can stimulate facet joint osteoarthritis with resultant osteophytes, further exacerbating the problem of narrowed space.

Facet instability and disc degeneration can produce a slippage of one vertebral body relative to the one below. This so-called degenerative spondylolisthesis further reduces the canal and foraminal dimensions. This type of slippage is distinguished from isthmic spondylolisthesis in which there is a defect of the pars interarticularis. (The pars interarticularis, or pars for short, is the part of a vertebra located between the inferior and superior articular processes of the facet joint. See https://orthopaedia.com/page/Spondylolysis-and-Spondylolisthesis) In degenerative spondylolisthesis there is no defect in the pars, and because the pars remains intact, the slip is often less than 25% of the width of the vertebral body and rarely greater than 50%. (With isthmic spondylolisthesis, where the pars interarticularis defects are often bilateral, slips greater than 50% are more commonly seen.)

The spinal cord terminates at roughly the L1 vertebral level, but the nerve roots that branch off the lower end of the spinal cord (the conus medullaris) remain within the central canal until they exit at their appropriate neural foramen. The nerves branching off beneath the termination of the spinal cord are said to resemble a horse's tail, hence the name cauda equina.

Thus, lumbar stenosis can compress all or part of the cauda equina. This compression can produce pain, paresthesia, and weakness in the pelvis and lower extremities. This can result in numbness in the legs and decreased walking distances.

PATIENT PRESENTATION

Patients with degenerative joint disease without stenosis are usually asymptomatic, but can report back pain or difficulty bending. If stenosis is present, patients may report buttock or lower extremity symptoms as well.

Osteophytes emanating from the vertebral bodies or facet joints may impinge on isolated nerve roots, causing pains or paresthesias suggestive of a disc herniation. Hypertrophy of the ligamentum flavum and disc prolapse additionally combine to narrow the spinal canal.

The back pain of lumbar spondylosis is often described as "mechanical", meaning that motion provokes the pain. Yet spondylosis can at times produce pain at rest as well: degeneration-induced instability of the vertebral bodies can initiate compensatory muscle spasm to limit motion and the pain from this muscle spasm might endure throughout the day, even at rest. This phenomenon can make diagnosis more difficult, as pain at rest normally suggests a cause outside of arthritis.

Lumbar stenosis can cause neurogenic claudication. (The word claudication comes from a Latin verb *claudicare,* meaning 'to limp', but in modern parlance refers to lower extremity pain and not a limp, per se.) The adjective "neurogenic" is used to distinguish this pattern of symptoms from vascular (or "classic") claudication, which is caused by peripheral arterial insufficiency. Both types of claudication are produced by ischemia: in neurogenic claudication the spinal nerve roots are ischemic, whereas in vascular claudication, the leg muscles themselves are deprived of blood flow.

One way to differentiate the two types of claudication is that neurogenic claudication alone can be relieved by bending over. Patients with neurogenic claudication report that riding a bicycle or walking while pushing a shopping cart produces surprisingly little pain, despite the exertion. Spinal flexion tends to maximally open the spinal canal, whereas extension of the spine as seen with upright standing tends to compress the central canal. (This is analogous to Phalen's maneuver compressing the carpal tunnel, with pressure relieved by holding the wrist in a neutral position.)

The location of the symptoms may be informative too. Neurogenic claudication usually causes symptoms proximally, primarily in the buttock and posterior thigh. Vascular claudication, mediated by decreased blood flow to the muscles, appears first distally in the calf.

On examination, patients with vascular claudication may show signs of arterial insufficiency such as cool, brittle, shiny skin on the legs, and weak or absent pulses. In contrast, patients with neurogenic claudication are more likely to have normal skin color, texture, and temperature in their lower extremities and normal palpable pulses.

Historically, students have been taught that vascular claudication can be identified by its "dose-dependent" symptoms, meaning that the pain of vascular claudication is initiated and worsened with movement and ameliorated by rest, in a crescendo/decrescendo pattern. By contrast, symptoms of neurogenic claudication were taught to be less related to the duration of activity and more to spinal position (flexion and extension). Although one recent study [doi: 10.1503/cjs.016512] found that the "classic symptom attributes used to differentiate neurogenic from vascular claudication are at best weakly valid independently," the constellation of symptoms can be a useful diagnostic guide.

OBJECTIVE EVIDENCE

Lab studies are usually not indicated unless there is concern for an infectious or neoplastic process. An electromyelogram (EMG) with nerve conduction studies can often help differentiate lower lumbar radiculopathy due to stenosis from peripheral neuropathy due to diabetes.

Radiographs in the setting of spondylosis (see Figures 5 and 6) may show disk-space narrowing, facet-joint hypertrophy, spondylolisthesis, end-plate sclerosis, and osteophytosis.

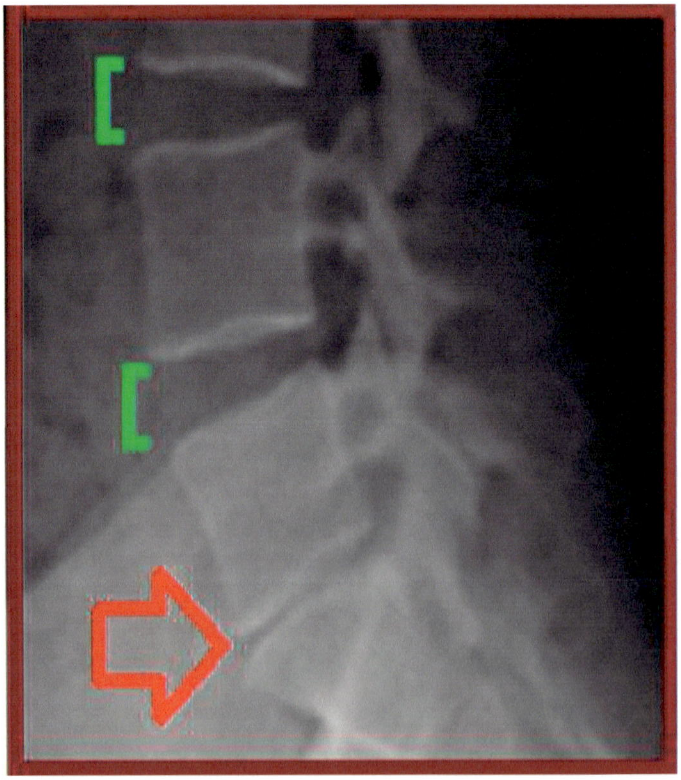

Figure 5: Lateral radiograph of the lumbar spine showing degenerative narrowing of the L5/S1 disc space (red arrow) contrasted to the normal space (shown in green) at the levels above. (Courtesy of https://doi.org/10.1155/2012/413913 Diagnostic Testing for Degenerative Disc Disease by Michael W. Hasz)

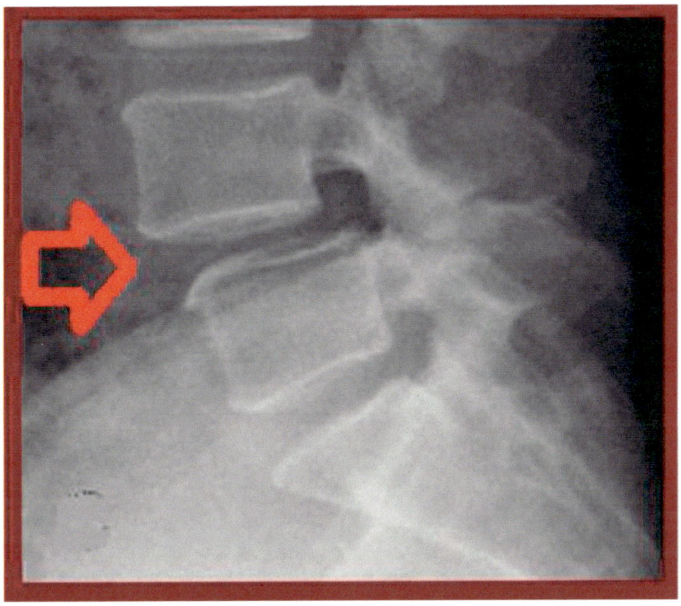

Figure 6: Lateral radiograph of the lumbar spine showing degenerative spondylolisthesis of L4-5 level (red arrow). (Courtesy of Minimally invasive versus traditional open transforaminal lumbar interbody fusion for the treatment of low-grade degenerative spondylolisthesis: a retrospective study. Sci Rep 10, 21851 (2020). https://doi.org/10.1038/s41598-020-78984-x)

Advanced imaging such as CT and MRI can confirm the diagnosis of spinal stenosis and can show both narrowing of the central canal and neural foramina. The central canal is considered stenotic when measured to have less than a 100 mm2 cross-sectional area or less than a 10 mm A-P diameter on CT scan.

CT is more sensitive for detecting bony abnormalities such as facet joint hypertrophy and osteophytes; MRI (see Figure 7) is more sensitive for detecting spinal stenosis from ligamentous hypertrophy and disc degeneration.

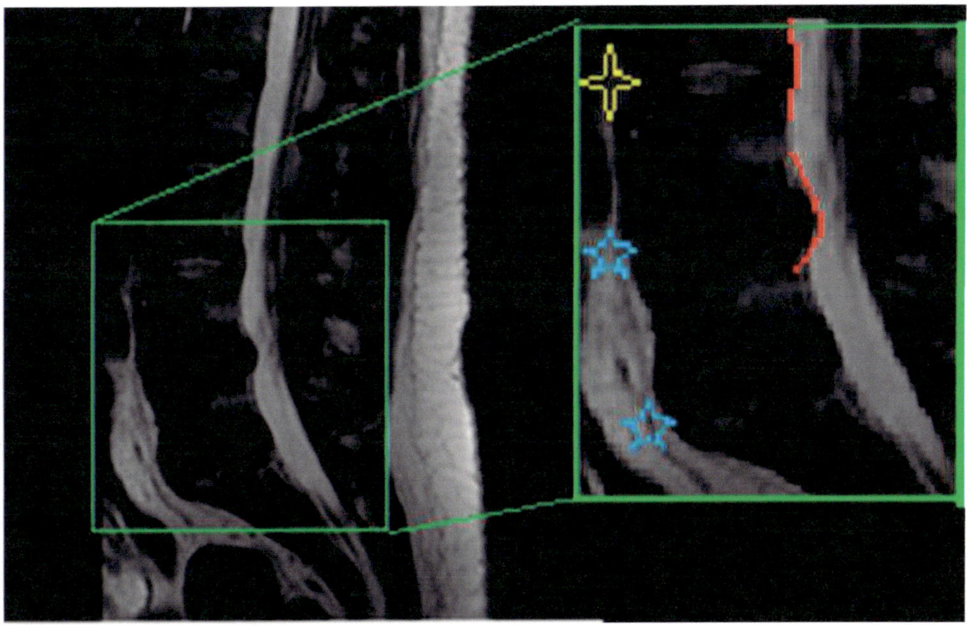

Figure 7: A sagittal T2-weighted MRI image demonstrating the darker discs at the L4-L5 and L5-S1 levels (blue stars), indicating dissection and degeneration, contrasted with the brighter signal within the L3-L4 disc, denoted by the yellow star. The normal posterior disc border at L3-L4 is contrasted with the protrusion of the L4-L5 disc (shown by red line). (Courtesy of https://doi.org/10.1155/2012/413913 Diagnostic Testing for Degenerative Disc Disease by Michael W. Hasz)

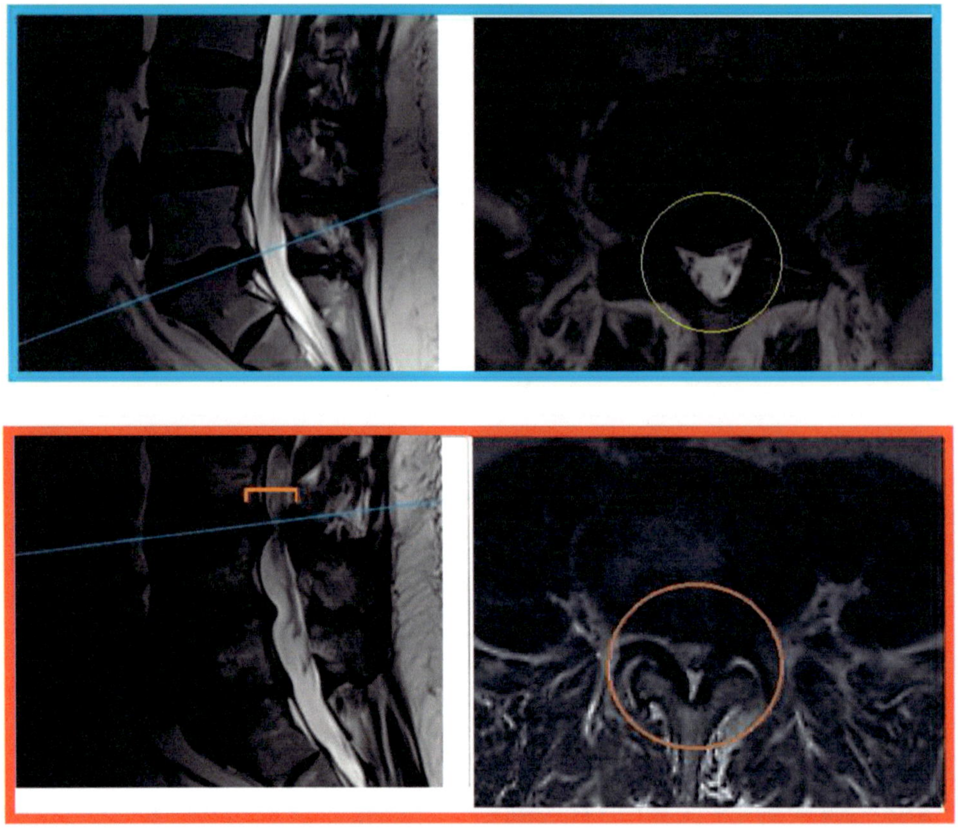

Figure 8: A matched pair of sagittal and axial views. The pair in the blue box above shows age-normal degenerative changes. The axial view shown at right is taken at the level of the blue line coursing through the disc in the figure at left. The space of the canal and recesses is shown by the yellow circle. Stenosis is seen below in the red box. In the sagittal view to the left, the decreased anterior-to-posterior space is outlined by the orange bracket. To the right, the smaller space of the stenotic canal and recesses is shown by the orange circle. (Images courtesy of Nader M. Hebela)

It is important to note that many people over the age of 60 may show signs of spinal stenosis on imaging even if they have no symptoms. Thus, although these imaging modalities are sensitive, they are not clinically specific.

Lastly, CT myelogram is an option for patients who cannot undergo an MRI. In a CT myelogram, dye is injected intrathecally. Radiographs and a CT scan are obtained to reveal neural structure impingement as well as bony abnormalities.

EPIDEMIOLOGY

Degenerative change in the spine is a universal phenomenon of aging. Approximately 10% of the adult population suffers from symptomatic lumbar spondylosis, with women and men affected equally. The peak incidence of seeking care for lumbar spondylosis occurs around the age of 65. Although degeneration increases with age, older people tend to be less active. These processes may offset, such that the objective increase in degenerative disease may not necessarily cause increased subjective symptoms. Lumbar spondylosis with stenosis most commonly occurs at the L4-5 level.

DIFFERENTIAL DIAGNOSIS

The differential diagnosis of lumbar spondylosis is based on the presenting symptoms. If the chief complaint is back pain, the following musculoskeletal diagnoses must be considered: muscular strains, disc disease, degenerative arthritis, inflammatory arthropathies, and less likely, infection and malignancy. (In patients at risk, osteoporotic compression fracture is also on the differential diagnosis.) If the chief complaint is claudication, the main diagnostic entities to consider are vascular insufficiency, diabetic neuropathy, and large central disc herniations.

Note also that back pain can have a non-musculoskeletal cause. Abdominal aortic aneurysms, gynecologic disorders such as endometriosis and tubal pregnancy, gastrointestinal disorders such as ulcers and pancreatitis, and kidney stones may present with back pain.

RED FLAGS

The compression of multiple nerves in the cauda equina often leads to unilateral or bilateral lower extremity pain and sensorimotor changes. Rarely, these changes can cause bowel/bladder dysfunction, manifest as incontinence or urinary retention (with overflow incontinence and increased post-void residuals).

Night pain can be present with lumbar degenerative disc disease/degenerative joint disease, as noted, but severe night pain – enough to wake the patient – especially if there are systemic complaints such as fever or weight loss, should raise suspicion of spinal infection or metastasis.

TREATMENT OPTIONS AND OUTCOMES

Needless to say, not all back pain requires medical treatment. Diagnostic investigations may discover incidental findings that are not the true cause of symptoms. Furthermore, surgical treatment is typically reserved for symptomatic neurologic compression, which manifests as lower extremity symptoms, and not isolated back pain.

If pain requires intervention, a non-operative approach is the best first option. Such treatment includes a period of *relative* (but not complete) rest, use of NSAIDs, hot or cold compresses, and physical therapy. Physical therapy is aimed at core strengthening and muscular rehabilitation. Stationary biking (and other exercises that incorporate lumbar flexion) are usually better tolerated by patients than exercises like walking or jogging that require lumbar extension.

Steroid injections and hyaluronic acid injections can be trialed prior to considering a more aggressive approach.

In cases of progressive neurologic deficits or unremitting and extremely debilitating pain, a patient may elect to proceed with a surgical procedure.

Laminectomy, which involves the partial or total excision of a lamina, may be used to remove osteophytes and fibrotic ligaments. Fusion can be performed in cases of spinal instability or degenerative spondylolisthesis (see Figure 9), although more recent studies are beginning to question the benefits of fusion versus laminectomy and decompression alone.

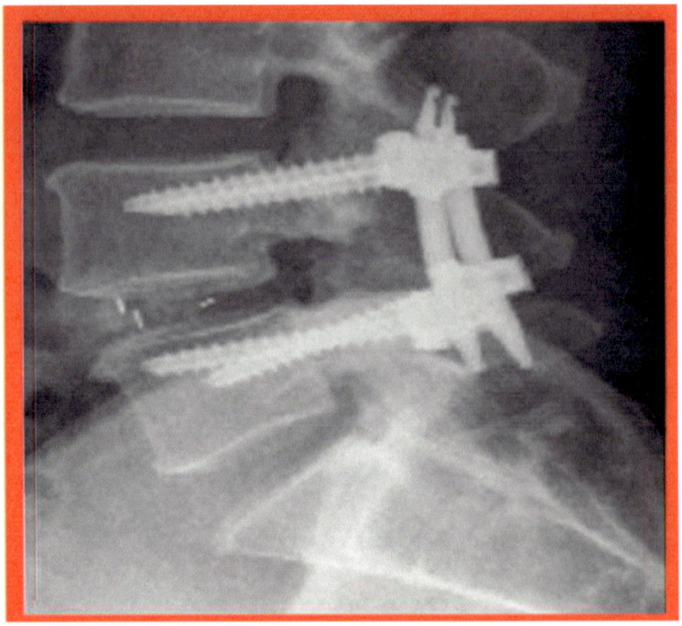

Figure 9: Lateral radiograph of the lumbar spine: Fusion of the degenerative L4-5 anterolisthesis shown above in Figure 6. (Courtesy of Minimally invasive versus traditional open transforaminal lumbar interbody fusion for the treatment of low-grade degenerative spondylolisthesis: a retrospective study. Sci Rep 10, 21851 (2020). https://doi.org/10.1038/s41598-020-78984-x)

Various types of decompressions can be performed, including laminectomy, laminotomy, or foraminotomy (Figure 10). The decision on which procedure to do depends on the location of the symptomatic neural compression.

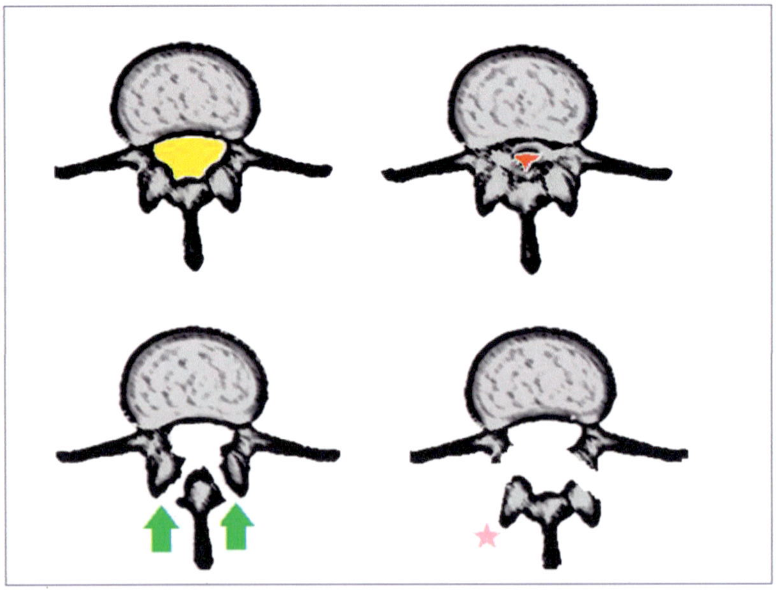

Figure 10: A schematic superior view of a normal lumbar vertebral body (top left) with a patent canal, shown in yellow. A similar view with lumbar spondylosis in which soft tissue and bony overgrowth along with disc protrusion produce a highly stenotic canal shown in red (top right). Shown at bottom left is a bilateral laminectomy (green arrows), with a wider decompression sacrificing the articular processes shown to the right (pink star). This more extensive resection provides greater decompression, but the absence of the facets necessitates the addition of surgical fusion to stabilize the spine.

Laminotomy, which removes only a small part of the lamina, can be used as an alternative to laminectomy.

Another alternative to laminectomy is interspinous distraction, although studies suggest that the benefits of this treatment do not persist over time.

Alternative therapies for lumbar spondylosis include yoga, transcutaneous electrical nerve stimulation (TENS), chiropractic, aromatherapy, acupuncture, and deep tissue massage.

Surgery has been associated with greater symptomatic improvement as compared to non-operative treatment at one to eight years, but this difference narrows through the years. Improvements in function and patient satisfaction are also noted with surgery, although recurrence of spinal stenosis adjacent to the level of decompression can occur. Reoperation and secondary procedures are needed in about 15% of cases. Common surgical complications include superficial and deep wound infections, dural tears, and blood loss requiring transfusion. Neurologic injuries, including sensory and motor dysfunction, are also possible complications but are seen less frequently.

RISK FACTORS AND PREVENTION

Age is the greatest risk factor in the development of lumbar degenerative spondylosis. Obesity (which increases the load on the spine), family history, and trauma or injury to the back are also known associations with these degenerative conditions as well as spinal stenosis. Specific occupations and sports that involve bending or heavy lifting can increase the risk of degenerative joint disease (DJD) and degenerative disc disease (DDD). Women are at a greater risk of developing DJD and spinal stenosis than are men. DJD, DDD, spondylolisthesis, spondylolysis, and congenitally shortened pedicles predispose an individual to spinal stenosis. The last scenario, known as congenital stenosis, usually becomes apparent in the 2nd through 4th decades. Shortened pedicles, though also seen in the general population, are a common feature of achondroplasia. Prior surgical interventions such as laminectomy and fusion are additional risk factors. Lastly, certain endocrinopathies and iatrogenic causes, such as Cushing's syndrome, Paget's disease, acromegaly, and exogenous steroid use, are associated with spinal stenosis.

Weight loss, proper technique when bending and lifting, and exercising good posture can help prevent the development of DJD and DDD. Physical activity that promotes core strengthening and back flexibility may also be beneficial.

MISCELLANY

Short-legged dog breeds, including dachshunds, basset hounds, corgis, and shih tzus, are very commonly affected by lumbar degenerative disc stenosis. Up to a quarter of dachshunds acquire the disease.

KEY TERMS

Spondylosis, degenerative disc disease (DDD), degenerative joint disease (DJD), facet joint arthritis, osteophytes, spinal stenosis, central stenosis, foraminal stenosis, neurogenic claudication, laminectomy, foraminotomy

SKILLS

Describe the process of disc and joint degeneration and understand how both conditions can lead to spinal stenosis. Differentiate neurogenic and vascular claudication. Identify the imaging findings associated with degenerative spondylosis.

CHAPTER 8.

SCHEUERMANN'S KYPHOSIS

Scheuermann's kyphosis is a rigid sagittal plane deformity within the thoracic, thoracolumbar, or lumbar spine. The cause of Scheuermann's kyphosis (often named as "Scheuermann's disease," or simply "Scheuermann's") is not known. This condition is characterized by uneven growth of the vertebrae in the sagittal plane. Posterior overgrowth results in wedging of the vertebrae and a rounded, hunched back that does not fully correct with active extension. Approximately 50% of cases of Scheuermann's kyphosis are associated with back pain.

STRUCTURE AND FUNCTION

Kyphosis refers to a convex curvature of the spine; the corresponding term, lordosis, refers to a concave curvature (see Figure 1). Normal thoracic kyphosis averages approximately 35 degrees with the cervical and lumbar spine both being lordotic.

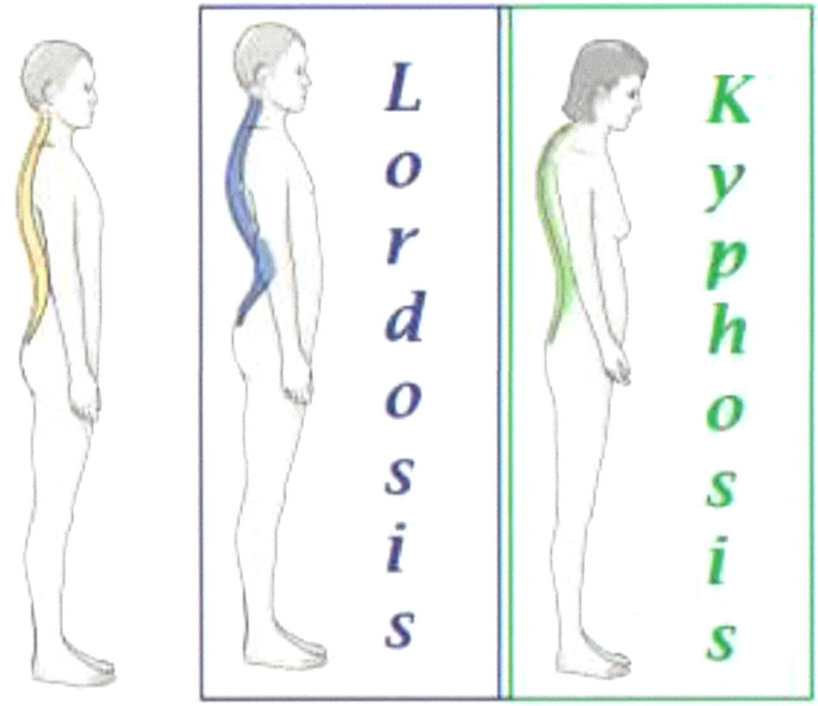

Figure 1: Normal sagittal plane alignment is shown at left, with excessive lordosis (blue arrow) and kyphosis (green arrow) shown in the center and right panels, respectively. (Image modified from Wikipedia)

Scheuermann's kyphosis is an increased amount of kyphosis (>45 degrees) and is defined radiographically. (Because some kyphosis is normally present, technically speaking this condition should be called "Scheuermann's hyperkyphosis.") The radiographic definition is a patient having three or more contiguous vertebrae with at least 5 degrees of anterior wedging. There are vertebral endplate abnormalities resulting in disc space narrowing that may be caused by an error in collagen aggregation. Schmorl's nodes, which are disc herniations into the vertebral endplate, are present.

The true etiology of Scheuermann's kyphosis is unknown but multiple theories exist. Scheuermann's theory was that the growth disturbance is due to osteonecrosis of the vertebral ring apophysis. This causes a growth arrest in the anterior vertebral body and radiographically is depicted by wedging. Schmorl's theory suggests disc material herniating through the vertebral end plate causes loss of height & ultimately the anterior wedging. Growth hormone abnormalities could possibly be a causative factor. Relative osteoporosis can lead to a compression deformity, thus causing the anterior vertebral wedging and increased kyphosis. There are possible genetic causes, as there is a high rate of heritability and an autosomal dominant inheritance pattern.

PATIENT PRESENTATION

The most evident clinical manifestation of Scheuermann's kyphosis comes with the physical exam. Patients will have increased kyphosis that is exacerbated with bending forward, (see Figure 2). The patients may also have compensatory hyperlordosis of the lumbar or cervical spine. This can lead to tightness in the hamstrings and iliopsoas muscles. Patients with more severe curves also have a higher incidence of back pain. Neurologic deficits, while rare, require a full neurologic exam.

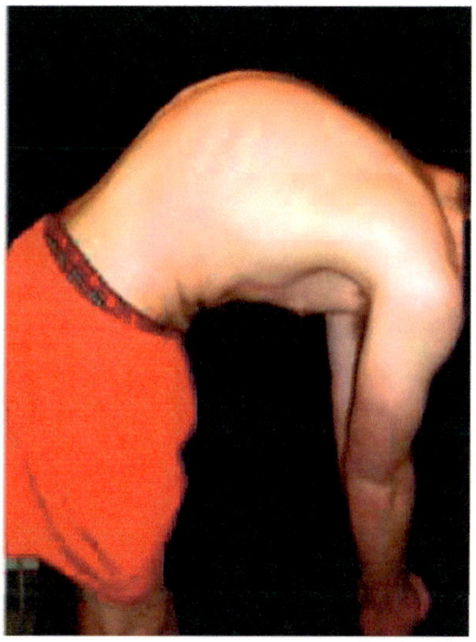

Figure 2: Clinical photograph of a 22-year-old male with a very extreme case of Scheuermann's disease. (courtesy Wikipedia)

OBJECTIVE EVIDENCE

After a patient's physical exam is worrisome for Scheuermann's kyphosis, an AP and lateral spine radiograph should be obtained (Figure 3).

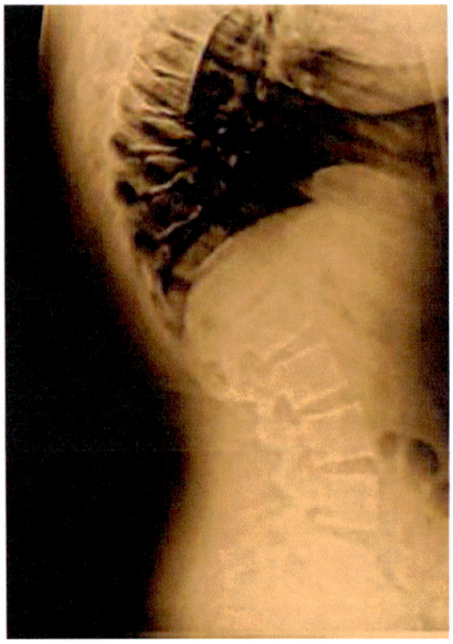

Figure 3: Lateral radiographs of a patient with Scheuermann's kyphosis (Case courtesy of Dr Bruno Lorensini, Radiopaedia.org, rID: 43740)

On the AP radiograph, the presence or absence of scoliosis should be noted. Lateral radiographs must be scrutinized to detect spondylolysis and spondylolisthesis.

Scheuermann's kyphosis is defined by a rigid thoracic hyperkyphosis greater than 45 degrees, associated with anterior wedging of three consecutive vertebrae measuring at least 5 degrees per vertebral body (Figure 4).

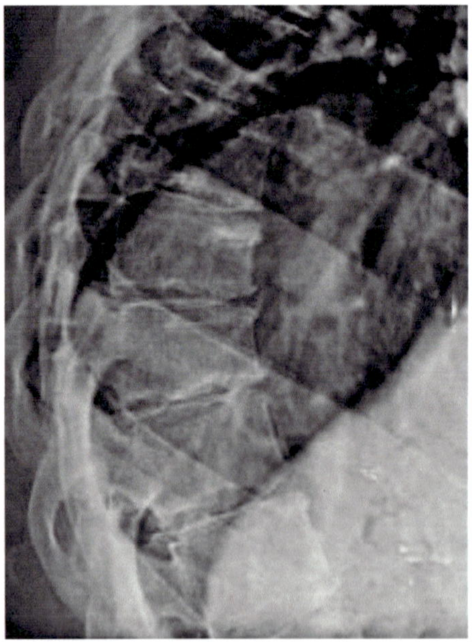

Figure 4: Wedging of the vertebral bodies. (Case courtesy of Dr Dalia Ibrahim, Radiopaedia.org, rID: 58862)

Disc space narrowing, endplate irregularities, and Schmorl's nodes can be noted on the lateral radiograph. Endplate irregularities are more common in thoracolumbar and lumbar Scheuermann's kyphosis compared to vertebral wedging.

Sagittal balance can be noted on the lateral radiograph by using the C7 plumb line and the posterior sacral vertical line.

The entire spine must be included on the x-ray as Scheuermann's kyphosis can extend all the way to the thoracolumbar regions. Thoracolumbar Scheuermann's is a far less common form, but is associated with increased back pain and more likely to be progressive.

A supine hyperextension lateral radiograph over a bolster may be obtained to differentiate Scheuermann's kyphosis from postural kyphosis. As opposed to postural kyphosis, Scheuermann's kyphosis is relatively inflexible on the hyperextension lateral radiograph.

MRI may be obtained at the discretion of the surgeon to identify disc herniations, spinal cord abnormalities, spondylolysis, spondylolisthesis, and spinal stenosis, among other spinal abnormalities. Any neurological deficit or symptom should be evaluated with an MRI.

EPIDEMIOLOGY

Scheuermann's kyphosis affects men and women equally, with a prevalence between 0.4%-10%. Scheuermann's kyphosis is the most common type of structural kyphosis in adolescents with a typical onset between the ages of 10-12. Thoracic Scheuermann's kyphosis is by far the most common, which is classified as a curve apex between T6-T8.

DIFFERENTIAL DIAGNOSIS

The main differentiation that must be made is between Scheuermann's kyphosis and postural kyphosis. Postural kyphosis will correct with extension, and radiographs will reveal the absence of anterior vertebral wedging.

Severe hyperkyphosis can be caused by vertebral compression fractures; this would be on the differential diagnosis for older females much more than in the pediatric or adolescent male population normally affected by Scheuermann's.

Congenital kyphosis may be found if vertebrae are malformed or fused. A congenital kyphosis in the absence of neurological disorders is rare.

Nutritional kyphosis can result from rickets, usually due to a vitamin D deficiency.

If there is lower back pain, spondylolysis and spondylolisthesis must be ruled out.

RED FLAGS

Any neurologic deficit or complaint should be evaluated with a full physical examination, radiograph, and advanced imaging. Back pain along with constitutional symptoms should be investigated fully. Spinal deformity may happen in the setting of malignancy, therefore imaging should be thoroughly evaluated by a radiologist as well as the ordering physician.

TREATMENT OPTIONS AND OUTCOMES

The treatment of mild to moderate (less than 50-80 degrees) Scheuermann's kyphosis is non-operative. Non-operative treatment includes stretching and physical therapy with routine radiographic follow up. Therapy and exercises include postural improvement, thoracic extensor strengthening, and core strengthening.

Bracing with an extension orthosis has been attempted (Figure 5). Bracing requires significant patient compliance with brace wear of 16-23 hours per day. As is the case with scoliosis, bracing is chosen not so much to affect a correction but to stop progression; thus, it is indicated only if there is remaining skeletal growth anticipated.

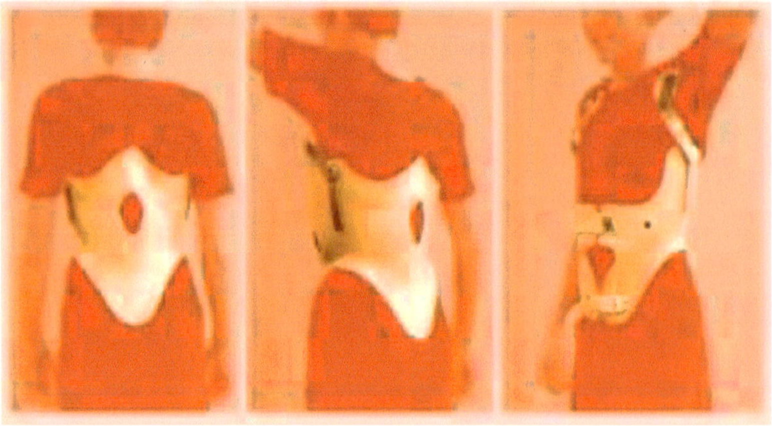

Figure 5: A thoraco-lumbar brace. (Photo modified from Wikipedia)

Operative treatment should be considered only in severe curves. Other indications for surgery include progressive deformity, neurologic deficit, spinal cord compression, and severe pain. Although there is no precise Cobb angle above which surgery is recommended, curves of 80 degrees or more in patients who have failed nonoperative treatment are usually indicated for surgery.

Surgery includes posterior instrumented spinal fusion with pedicle screw fixation (Figure 6). Anterior surgery is much less common with improvements in posterior surgical intervention. With severe, rigid curves posterior (Ponte) osteotomies may be performed. About 5 to 10 degrees of correction is anticipated with each posterior osteotomy performed. More aggressive osteotomies (pedicle subtraction or vertebral column resection) can be used with increased risk of complications. Intraoperative neuromonitoring is the standard of care in patients with spinal deformity.

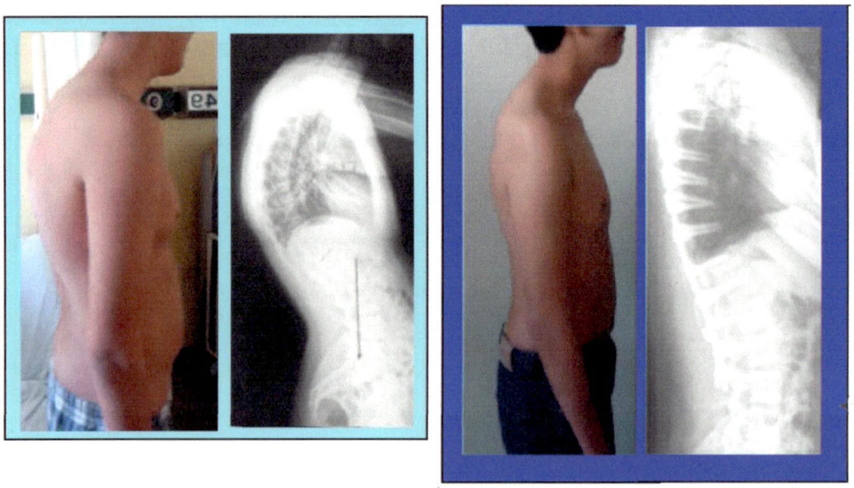

Figure 6: Clinical photos and lateral x-rays of a patient with Scheuermann's kyphosis before and after posterior instrumented spinal fusion. (Courtesy Surgical treatment of Scheuermann´s disease by the posterior approach. Case series. Coluna/Columna, 14(1), 14-17. https://doi.org/10.1590/S1808-1851201514010R120)

Patients with curves less than 60 degrees typically have a benign course and a good clinical outcome with observation alone. Patients with kyphosis greater than 100 degrees have clinically significant impairment in pulmonary function.

The Scoliosis Research Society and Harms Study Group both reported an overall complications rate of approximately 15% in Scheuermann's Kyphosis.

Neurologic complications with posterior spinal fusion have a reported rate of 0.6-0.8%, which is slightly higher than the rates in idiopathic scoliosis. There is conflicting evidence on whether combined anterior/posterior procedures have higher neuromonitoring changes compared to posterior only procedures.

Proximal and distal junctional kyphosis are complications that can be mitigated by selecting appropriate fusion levels, avoiding overcorrection >50% of original curve, construct choice, and correcting sagittal balance.

MISCELLANEOUS

While the natural history of Scheuermann's kyphosis tends to be benign, patients are more likely to pursue jobs that require less strenuous physical activity. Also, there is a cosmetic deformity. In all, there are important psychosocial considerations beyond the medical aspects of the condition.

KEY TERMS

Kyphosis, Schmorl's node

SKILLS

Evaluate lateral x-rays of the spine and identify abnormal alignment. Identify signs of abnormal spinal alignment.

CHAPTER 9.

SPINAL INFECTION

Infections of the spine can occur in several adjacent yet anatomically distinct locations: the vertebral bodies, the intervertebral discs and the epidural space (see Figure 1). Infection of the vertebral bodies is termed "osteomyelitis," as it would be any other bone. Disc and epidural space infections are denoted as "discitis" and "spinal epidural abscess" respectively. In general, the most commonly implicated organisms are bacterial, but spinal infection can also be caused by mycobacterium, fungi or, less commonly, viruses.

Spinal infections are relatively rare but are clinically important as they may cause significant morbidity and mortality – especially damage to the spinal cord and nerve roots that manifest as pain and dysfunction. Accordingly, suspected spinal infection requires urgent medical attention.

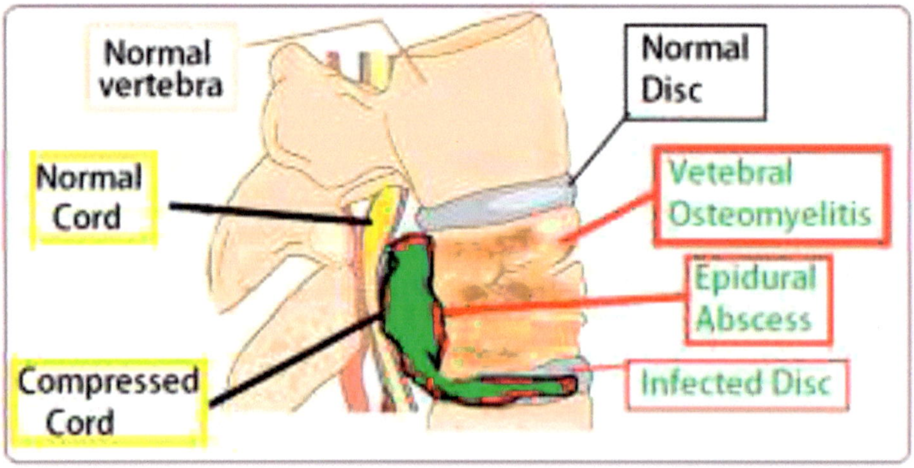

Figure 1: Sagittal drawing of the spine showing the three areas for potential infection: the vertebral body, the intervertebral disc and the epidural space. (Modified from Spinal Epidural Abscess: A Review Highlighting Early Diagnosis and Management. JMA J. 2020;3(1):29-40)

STRUCTURE AND FUNCTION

The primary anatomic regions of the spine that are susceptible to infection include the vertebral bodies, the intervertebral disc, and the epidural space. These distinct anatomic regions have different blood supplies and therefore different capacities to spread infections. Of the three, the epidural space is most vascular, followed by the bone; the intervertebral disc is the least vascular.

The term vertebral osteomyelitis refers to an infection localized to the bones of the vertebral column. Vertebral osteomyelitis is usually seeded from a hematogenous source, that is, pathogens circulating in the blood which spread to the bones of the spine. If the vertebral bodies become infected, they can lose their structural integrity and collapse, leading to deformity.

Discitis refers to an infection of the intervertebral disc space. If both the disc space and the adjacent vertebral body are infected, as is common with bacterial infections, the term "spondylodiscitis" may be used.

An epidural abscess is a contained collection of purulent fluid in the area between the dura mater and the vertebral bone (see Figure 2). The epidural space contains arteries and veins which can be compressed by the abscess. An abscess can cause septic thrombophlebitis, which can further impede blood flow. A larger abscess can compress the spinal cord and nerve roots directly.

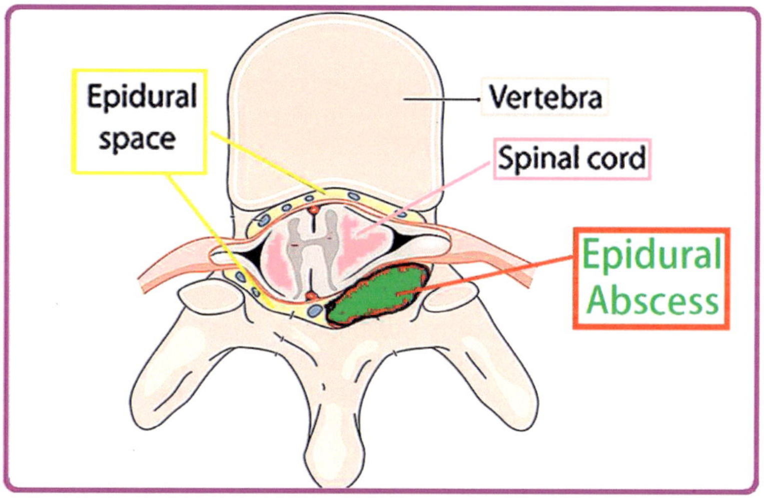

Figure 2: Drawing of an axial view of the spine, showing a posterior epidural abscess. This posterior abscess creates a mass effect that indents the spinal cord from behind. There is also compression of the vessels within the epidural space. (Image courtesy of Spinal Epidural Abscess: A Review Highlighting Early Diagnosis and Management. JMA J. 2020;3(1):29-40)

Although osteomyelitis, discitis and spinal epidural abscesses refer to discrete infection patterns, these conditions can overlap when there is a progression of a single infectious focus. For example, osteomyelitis can extend posteriorly to form an epidural abscess or it might spread to the adjacent intervertebral disc and vertebral body, causing spondylodiscitis.

The etiology of most spinal infections is usually seeding of the spine from a distant source of infection via the bloodstream, (so-called hematogenous spread).

The age of the patient influences the specific location prone to infection, as the blood supply to the spine changes with age. In children, the nucleus pulposus of each intervertebral disc is well-vascularized. Thus, in children, infection from a distal origin will spread to the nucleus pulposus preferentially. In adults, the nucleus pulposus is avascular, whereas the vertebral bodies and end plates have a relatively higher volume/low velocity blood flow. Therefore, in the adult, streaming bacteria are more apt to land in the bone.

Beyond arterial hematogenous spread, other modes of infection of the spine include direct inoculation of the spine and contiguous spread from adjacent soft tissues. Direct inoculation may occur due to iatrogenic injury during surgery or from penetrating trauma. An infected sacral decubitus ulcer or retropharyngeal/retroperitoneal abscess might be the source of contiguous spread. Contiguous spread may also be the result of a lung infection or psoas muscle abscess which, if left untreated, can extend into the nearby vertebral bodies.

Vertebral osteomyelitis affects the lumbar spine in a majority of cases. The thoracic spine is affected in about 35% of cases and the cervical spine in about 10% of cases. *S.aureus* is the most common bacteria responsible for vertebral osteomyelitis accounting for 50% or more of cases; *S.epidermis* is the second most common organism. Other less common organisms include gram negative bacteria (often originating from septic genitourinary or respiratory tract infections), pseudomonas (most common in intravenous drug users), salmonella (as seen in patients with sickle cell disease), and Brucella (common in countries where unpasteurized sheep, goat, or camel milk is consumed).

Vertebral osteomyelitis leads to abscess formation in about 20% of cases. Spinal epidural abscesses are almost always found due to progression of adjacent osteomyelitis or discitis.

PATIENT PRESENTATION

The general complaints most often elicited on history from patients with an infectious diseases of the spine include severe and debilitating back pain for more than a week, fever, and malaise. In addition, it is important to elicit any relevant predisposing factors for spinal infection (see *Risk Factors* below), as this may help aid in forming the differential diagnosis. Any decline in motor or sensory function requires further diagnostic imaging and laboratory studies.

The diagnosis of disc space infection in young children can be especially challenging given their limited ability to articulate their symptoms. Clinical clues in toddlers include a refusal to sit or walk and resistance to physical activity. In addition, painful limping, change in appetite, fever, and abdominal or back pain can be consistent with discitis.

In older children or adolescents, focal back pain and point tenderness are the usual (and non-specific) findings for spinal infection.

Vertebral osteomyelitis can present with an acute, subacute, or chronic disease course, most often in an adult 60 years of age or older. Back pain is the most common initial symptom, and is present in over 85% of cases. Fever, however, is a less reliable finding, occurring in only about half or less of cases. The absence of fever can be misleading, as patients are often taking NSAID analgesics that may suppress fever as well.

Patients with a spinal epidural abscess most often have one or more predisposing risk factors or conditions such as diabetes, immunodeficiency syndromes, intravenous drug use, prior spine surgery, malnutrition, and recent systemic infection.

Spinal epidural abscess can present with a classic triad of fever, spinal pain, and neurologic deficits, but the complete triad is found concurrently in only a fraction of patients. The most common symptom is severe back pain, which occurs in the majority of patients. Fever is present in only about 50% of patients. While neurologic deficits are the most feared complication of spinal epidural abscess, only about a third of patients will present with neurologic symptoms or exam findings. Nonetheless, it is important to inquire about numbness, paresthesia, bowel, bladder and sexual dysfunction, and lower extremity motor weakness.

OBJECTIVE EVIDENCE

The diagnosis of spinal infection is challenging given the nonspecific signs and symptoms. Thus, spinal infection should always be included on the differential for any patient with known risk factors or with constitutional symptoms suggestive of infection.

Acute phase reactants, erythrocyte sedimentation rate (ESR), C-reactive protein (CRP), and procalcitonin (PCT) levels are elevated in >80% of patients with disc space infection or vertebral osteomyelitis. Note, however, these lab tests could be elevated for a multitude of reasons. Thus, ESR, CRP and PCT are good screening tests in patients with symptoms concerning for spinal infection but do not establish the diagnosis themselves. Rather, elevated acute phase reactant values suggest the need for further investigation with advanced imaging.

Despite its low specificity, the CRP trend can be used to monitor for effectiveness of treatment: baseline levels are expected to decrease as the infection is cleared.

The white blood count (WBC) is only elevated in about half of patients with vertebral osteomyelitis or disc space infection.

Blood cultures and urine cultures are also important in identifying a potential infection source and thus guiding treatment, though cultures are positive in only about 50% of patients. However, it is important to obtain cultures in patients suspected of having a spinal infection, as positive results would preclude the need for more invasive diagnostic procedures to identify the causative organism and antibiotic sensitivities. When the causative organism is not identified by blood culture, a vertebral body biopsy may be needed.

Plain radiographs are routinely obtained, though they will often not show any changes until at least 2 weeks after infection. Some of the early findings for spondylodiscitis are loss of vertebral body architecture and paraspinous soft tissue swelling. Later findings include disc space narrowing, endplate erosion or vertebral body collapse, which begin to appear 10-21 days after the onset of infection. CT scans (Figure 3) are similar to what plain radiographs may show, only they are more sensitive for earlier changes in the bone.

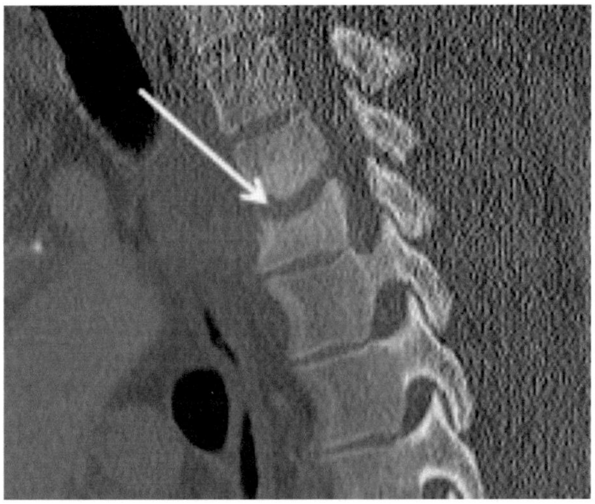

Figure 3: A sagittal CT demonstrates osseous destruction of the endplates at the T2–T3 level (arrow) with reactive sclerosis of the adjacent vertebral bodies in a patient with pyogenic spondylodiscitis. (Image courtesy Imaging spinal infection https://doi.org/10.1016/j.jrid.2016.03.001)

Radiographs have a very limited role in diagnosing an isolated spinal epidural abscess, as the collection usually cannot be visualized at all.

MRI (see Figure 4) with contrast is the gold standard imaging modality, with approximately 95% sensitivity and specificity for spondylodiscitis. Findings include a decreased signal intensity in the focus of infection within the vertebral bodies and discs on T1-weighted images, increased vertebral body enhancement on T2-weighted images, and contrast (often gadolinium) enhancement of paraspinal and epidural processes.

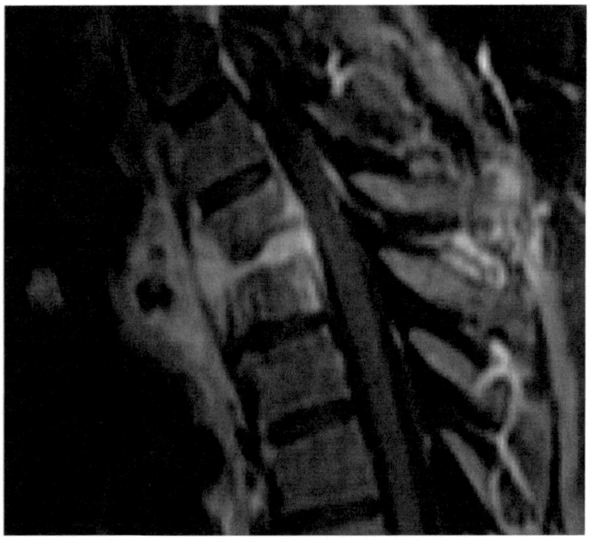

Figure 4: Sagittal T1-weighted fat-saturated post contrast images of the patient shown in the figure above demonstrate enhancement of the intervertebral disk space and adjacent vertebral bodies at the T2–T3 level. (Image courtesy of Imaging spinal infection https://doi.org/10.1016/j.jrid.2016.03.001)

MRI is particularly useful for visualizing the epidural space (Figure 5). Epidural abscesses tend to have low signal on T1-weighted images and high or intermediate intensity on T2-weighted ones.

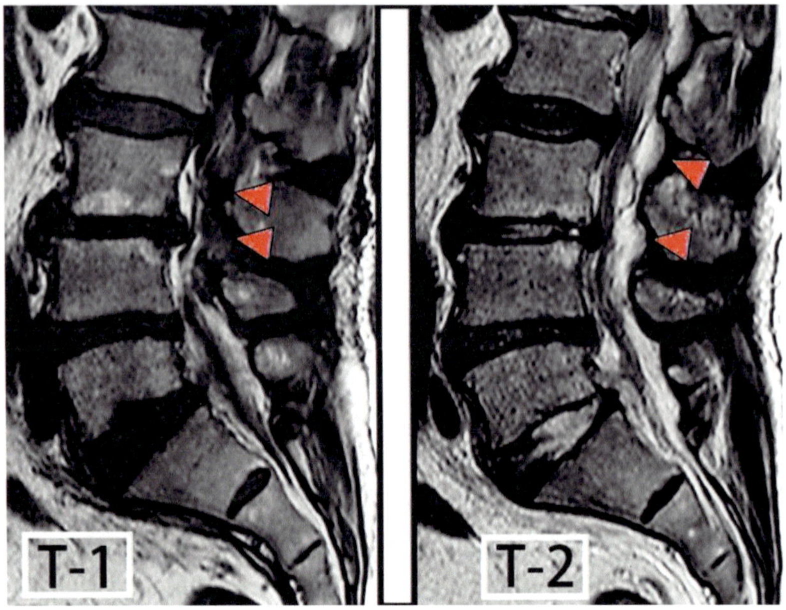

Figure 5: Sagittal T1-weighted, T2-weighted images of the lumbar spine showing a lumbar epidural abscess. The T1-weighted image to the left shows low signal intensity whereas the T2-weighted image shows high signal intensity. (Image courtesy of Spinal Epidural Abscess: A Review Highlighting Early Diagnosis and Management. JMA J. 2020;3(1):29-40.)

Importantly, MRI can help rule out other items on the differential diagnosis list such as malignancy.

For patients who cannot undergo MRI, technetium bone scan is a reasonable alternative for the diagnosis of spondylodiscitis, but it is less sensitive and far less specific.

More invasive diagnostic procedures may be required in patients with clinical and radiographic evidence of osteomyelitis with negative blood/urine cultures, as identifying the organism is critical in choosing the appropriate antibiotic. The gold standard for these patients is a CT-guided biopsy with culture and histopathology (see Figure 6). This method of obtaining a culture reveals a higher diagnostic yield relative to blood culture, but is obviously more invasive with a higher rate of complications. Histopathology of the biopsy specimen may provide evidence of more rare infections (brucellosis or tuberculosis) characterized by granuloma formation. If the first biopsy is non-conclusive an additional biopsy is recommended as it increases the likelihood of identifying an infectious agent. As a last resort diagnostically, an open biopsy would be indicated in patients with a negative CT-guided biopsy in the setting of a very high suspicion for infection.

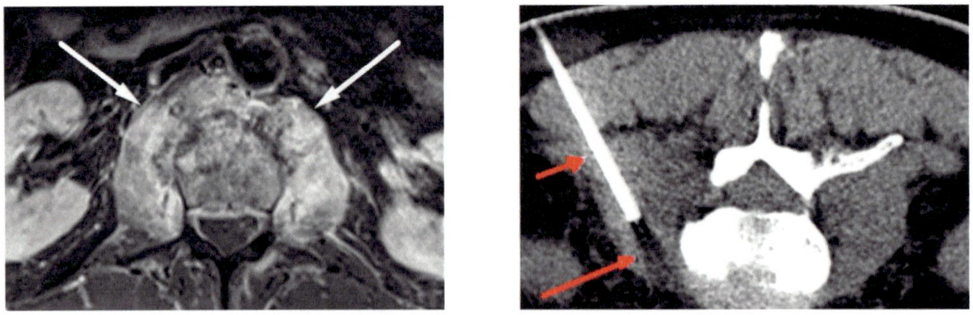

Figure 6: An abscess (white arrows) is identified in the left psoas muscle in the MRI image to the left. A CT-guided biopsy of the psoas abscess (red arrows) is shown in the figure to the right. (Image courtesy of CT-Guided Biopsy in Suspected Spondylodiscitis – The Association of Paravertebral Inflammation with Microbial Pathogen Detection https://doi.org/10.1371/journal.pone.0146399)

EPIDEMIOLOGY

Spinal infections are relatively rare conditions. Discitis is estimated to occur in 3/100,000 pediatric patients annually, most often in children younger than 5 years old, males more than females.

Isolated disc space infections in adults are rare; the most common cause of discitis is progression of adjacent vertebral osteomyelitis (spondylodiscitis).

The incidence of vertebral osteomyelitis is approximately 2/100,000 per year. However, the incidence is increasing, likely as a consequence of the rising prevalence of intravascular devices and surgical procedures (usually spinal surgery), immunosuppressive medications, chronic diseases (e.g., diabetes), and the aging population.

Spinal epidural abscess is seen in fewer than 1/100,000 people per year.

DIFFERENTIAL DIAGNOSIS

The differential diagnosis for spinal infection includes malignancy (primary or metastatic), inflammatory arthritis, vertebral compression fracture and visceral infection/abscess. Ordinary degenerative spondylosis and disc disease, owing to their prevalence, must also be considered.

While there are features on history and physical exam that can help sort this differential diagnosis list, the nonspecific nature of the symptoms in spinal infection often leads to a reliance on objective findings such as imaging and laboratory tests.

RED FLAGS

The most feared complications of spinal infections are permanent neurologic damage and sepsis. Thus, the major red flag symptoms include any neurologic deficits suggesting involvement of the spinal cord or any hemodynamic instability or severe systemic symptoms concerning for sepsis. Therefore, a thorough neurological exam is warranted in all patients that exhibit these signs and symptoms since it helps increase our index of suspicion.

TREATMENT OPTIONS AND OUTCOMES

Because one of the complications of infection includes hemodynamic instability, fluid resuscitation and intravenous broad-spectrum antibiotics (such as vancomycin and a third-generation cephalosporin) should be given to any patient presenting with signs of sepsis– even prior to confirmation of the offending microbe.

Ideally, blood cultures are drawn before antibiotics are given, as a culture provides not only a general diagnosis but is critical for tailoring the appropriate antibiotic treatment. In the stable patient with a suspected disc space infection, vertebral osteomyelitis, or spondylodiscitis, antibiotics should ideally be withheld until a culture-proven diagnosis is made.

The specific antibiotic will depend upon the causative organism, but patients will typically require 6-12 weeks of antibiotics. Potentially useful non-operative adjuncts include bed rest to reduce stress on the spine, analgesics for pain, and bracing to help reduce pain and prevent potential spinal deformity.

The majority of cases of isolated spondylodiscitis without abscess formation do not require surgery: antibiotics and occasionally bracing will suffice.

If a spinal epidural abscess is present, urgent surgical decompression might be required, especially in the presence of any neurological deficits. Traditionally, surgical decompression has been indicated for all cases of epidural abscess formation. However, more recent data has suggested that it may be reasonable to treat patients with antibiotics alone if three main criteria are fulfilled: 1) the abscess is small, 2) no neurologic deficits are present and 3) a microbiologic diagnosis can be made via blood culture or CT-guided aspiration. Needless to say, in cases that do not meet those criteria, or fail to respond to antibiotic treatment, surgical drainage with debridement of the infected tissues is recommended, especially given the morbidity associated with incompletely treated epidural infections.

After surgical drainage of an abscess, a post-operative course of antibiotics for 2 to 4 weeks is thought to be sufficient if there is no bony involvement. On the other hand, if the bone is infected as well, the antibiotic treatment should be extended to at least 6 weeks and sometimes even to 12 weeks.

Complications of isolated spondylodiscitis without abscess formation include narrowing of the disc space, spinal deformity, and persistent back pain. Overall, there is an 80% success rate with non-operative treatment, but morbidity and mortality of infections increase with age. The mortality rate is relatively low at <5%.

The complication rate and prognosis are less favorable for spinal epidural abscess. There is an approximate 15% incidence of permanent neurological damage from either direct compression or infarction of the spinal cord. The mortality rate of spinal epidural abscesses is about 5%. Ultimately, the most important predictor of neurologic outcome is the patient's neurologic status immediately prior to surgery, highlighting the importance of early and accurate diagnosis of this condition.

RISK FACTORS AND PREVENTION

There are several risk factors associated with the development of a spinal infection. These include immunodeficiency or immunosuppression (diabetes, medications, primary immunodeficiency syndrome), intravenous drug use, increasing age, malignancy, trauma, existing degenerative spine disease, malnutrition, obesity, and recent systemic infection. Some of these risk factors are amenable to modification, often only with great effort and good luck.

Two other risk factors are worthy of special mention: tuberculosis (TB) and prior spine surgery.

Although tuberculosis is uncommon in the United States (with fewer than 3 cases per 100,000 persons), it is highly prevalent in other parts of the world. Thus, spinal tuberculosis should be considered and excluded in patients coming from countries where tuberculosis is endemic. Approximately 5% of all TB patients have spine involvement (see Figure 7). A chest x-ray should be ordered for any patients in which TB is a possibility, as late diagnosis is associated with severe and irreversible kyphosis (even after successful treatment).

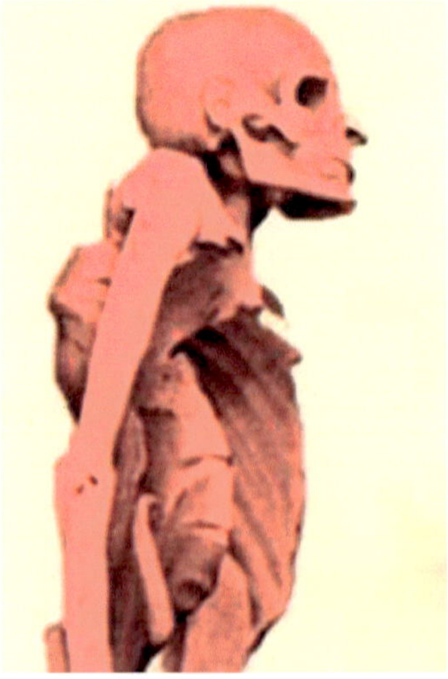

Figure 7: Tuberculosis of the spine in an Egyptian mummy from approximately 1000 B.C.E. (Courtesy of Wikipedia)

Brucellosis, uncommon in the USA, is more prevalent in parts of the world where people drink unpasteurized sheep, goat, or camel milk. Brucella, like other bacteria, may be identified by routine blood cultures and is not readily apparent on most radiographic tests unless signs of osteomyelitis are already present.

Postoperative spine infections are relatively rare but can have catastrophic sequelae. Thus, they must be detected as quickly as possible. Post-operative patients, especially if there is implanted hardware, should be monitored closely with urgent treatment initiated when signs suggesting infection are present. Wound drainage is the most common presentation but often the presentation is more subtle. A good heuristic to detect a post-operative infection is to pay attention to the pattern of pain. In general, post-operative pain should decrease as time from surgery passes. Pain that increases with time is therefore suspicious.

MISCELLANEOUS

Tuberculosis of the spine is known as Pott's Disease (see Figure 8).

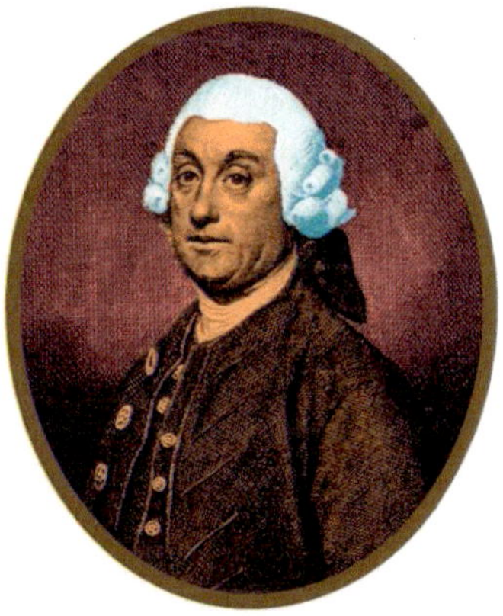

Figure 8: Percivall Pott was an English surgeon who described spinal tuberculosis, hence the eponym "Pott's disease." In 1769, he published one of the first books on orthopaedic surgery, Some Few Remarks upon Fractures and Dislocations.

KEY TERMS

Vertebral osteomyelitis, disc space infection, discitis, spondylodiscitis, spinal epidural abscess

SKILLS

Understand the anatomic and pathophysiologic differences between vertebral osteomyelitis, discitis, and spinal epidural abscess. Perform a targeted history and physical exam with special attention to red flags concerning for spinal cord involvement or sepsis. Identify the appropriate labs and imaging studies that will help confirm the diagnosis of spinal infection.

CHAPTER 10.

SPINAL TRAUMA & SPINAL CORD INJURY: GENERAL PRINCIPLES

Injuries to the spine – the vertebral bodies, their surrounding soft tissues, and the spinal cord itself – can cause devastating neurological consequences. Rapid evaluation of any patient with potential spinal trauma is crucial to rule out damage to the spinal cord and nerve roots. Even without neurological involvement, spinal injuries can be very painful and possibly disabling. In this section, the general principles of spinal trauma will be presented. A selection of more specific traumatic spinal conditions will be discussed in a separate chapter.

STRUCTURE AND FUNCTION

The spinal column is divided into four main parts: cervical, thoracic, lumbar, and sacral (Figure 1). Twenty-four vertebral bodies (7 cervical, 12 thoracic, 5 lumbar) extend from the foramen magnum at the skull to the sacrum at the pelvis.

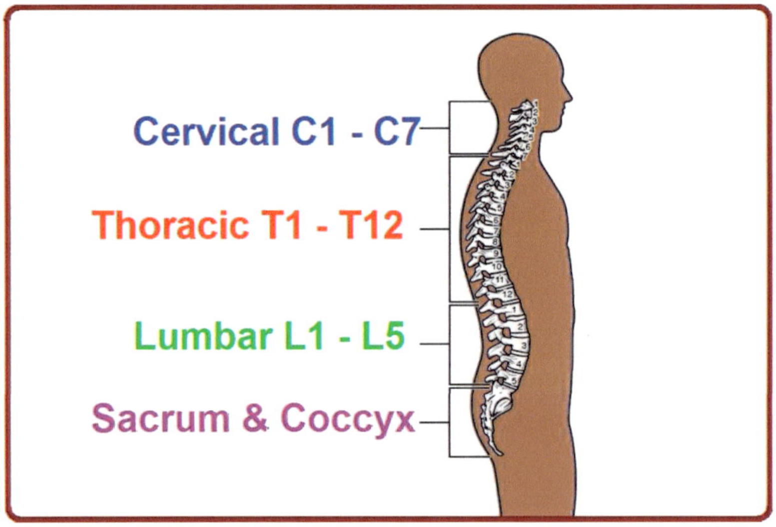

Figure 1: The regions of the spinal column. (From https://openstax.org/books/anatomy-and-physiology/pages/7-3-the-vertebral-column)

The first cervical vertebra (C1) is known as the atlas, and the second (C2) is known as the axis. The atlas articulates with the occiput of the head above and the axis below. The morphology of the atlas and the axis differ markedly from the other vertebrae below them. The atlas has no vertebral body and no spinous process. Rather, there are lateral masses connected by anterior and posterior arches. The C2 vertebra has an odontoid process (also known as the dens) which is a peg or protuberance that enters the C1 body, creating the atlanto-axial joint for rotation of the head (see Figure 2).

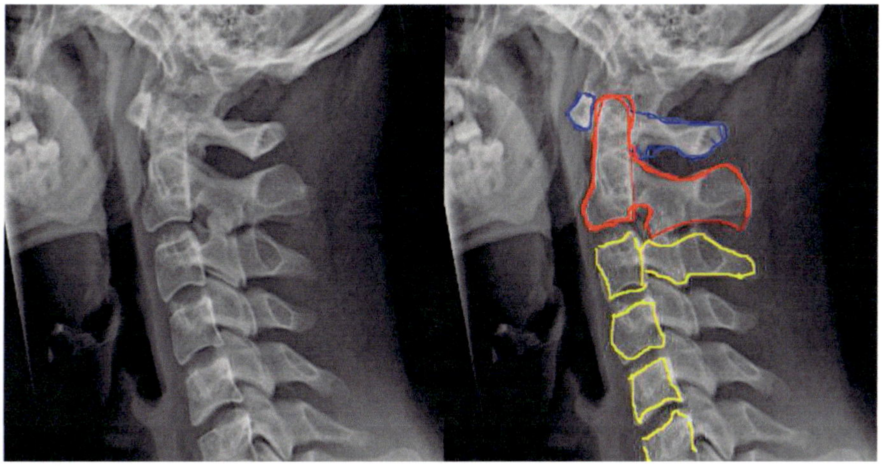

Figure 2: A lateral x-ray of the cervical spine, with an annotated view at right. In this annotation, C1 is outlined in blue, C2 in red (showing the projection of the odontoid into C1), and the lower cervical vertebrae in yellow. (Courtesy of Wikimedia.org)

The vertebral bodies are draped front and back by the anterior and posterior longitudinal ligaments, respectively. The ligamentum flavum covers the posterior aspect of the spinal canal and connects the lamina while the interspinal and intertransverse ligaments connect the spinous processes and transverse processes of adjacent vertebrae, respectively. Discs are situated between each vertebral body to act as cushions.

The spinal cord travels through the spinal canal from the foramen magnum to (approximately) the caudal aspect of the L1 vertebral body. It is bordered in the front by the vertebral bodies, to the sides by the pedicles, and to the back by the laminae.

At each vertebral level, the dorsal and ventral rami come together to create the nerve roots, which exit the spine through the lateral foramen.

At that point, the cord forms the conus medullaris and gives off a collection of nerve roots called the cauda equina (as this collection is said to resemble a horse's tail). These peripheral nerves travel through the spinal canal until their point of exit at a neural foramen. In the cervical spine, the vertebral arteries pass through the transverse foramina before entering the foramen magnum.

Different portions of the spinal column have different propensities for injury. Most of the thoracic spine down to T10, for example, is relatively protected during trauma by its articulation with the inherently stable rib cage. On the other hand, the thoracolumbar region (T11-L2) has more flexibility and mobility, which enhances its daily utility, but makes the region more prone to injury in trauma. Likewise, at each of the junctions between regions –occipitocervical, cervicothoracic, thoracolumbar, and lumbosacral– mobility is maximized at the cost of stability.

PATIENT PRESENTATION

Spinal trauma has a bimodal age distribution. Younger patients typically present after high-energy trauma such as motor vehicle collisions. Geriatric patients are injured by low-energy mechanisms such as falls in the setting of osteoporosis and degenerative changes in the spine.

There are approximately one million spinal fractures each year in the US. Of those, approximately 75% involve the thoracolumbar spine. Spinal cord injuries occur far less frequently, with about 10,000 new cases per year. Approximately half of these cases involve the cervical region, with the remaining half divided between the thoracic or lumbar regions. The level of function after spinal cord injury can be assessed on physical examination by motor and sensory testing (see Tables 1 and 2) and is more commonly assessed using the American Spinal Injury Association (ASIA) scoring system (see Figure 3).

Root	Motor Function	Sensory area
C5	Elbow flexion	Lateral shoulder
C6	Wrist extension	Dorsum of thumb and index finger
C7	Elbow extension	Dorsum of middle finger
C8	Finger flexors	Dorsum of ring and small finger
T1	Finger abductors	Medial forearm

Table 1: Upper extremity root levels.

Root	Motor Function	Sensory area
L2	Hip flexors	Anterior mid-thigh
L3	Knee extension	Anterior knee
L4	Ankle extension (dorsiflexion)	Medial leg
L5	Long toe extension	Medial dorsum foot
S1	Ankle plantar flexion	Lateral plantar foot

Table 2: Lower extremity root levels.

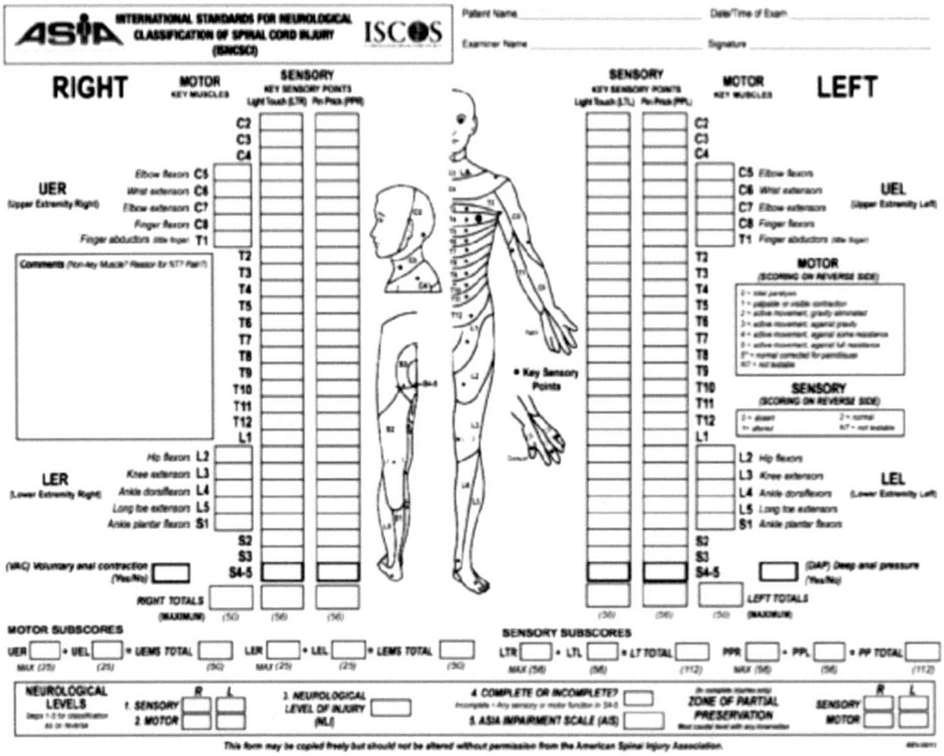

Figure 3: The 2019 revision of the International Standards for Neurological Classification of Spinal Cord Injury. (Reproduced with permission of the American Spinal Injury Association (ASIA))

As a rule, the higher the level of injury, the greater the functional loss. If the functional injury is at the C6 level, wrist extension and supination are intact; thus, patients can often feed themselves. When C7 function is retained, patients can power a manual wheelchair or perform transfers from chair to bed, since they have persevered triceps function. T1 level function, which powers the hand intrinsic muscles, is needed to have full manual dexterity. Injuries in the lumbar spine cause lower extremity dysfunction and urinary/fecal continence.

Cord injury can further be categorized as complete or incomplete. Incomplete injury leads to some measure of voluntary distal motor and/or perianal sensation. Neurological impairment can be classified using the American

Spinal Injury Association Impairment Scale (see Table 3). Complete spinal cord injury can only be defined once the patient is no longer in spinal shock, a point defined by the return of the normal bulbocavernosus reflex arc.

American Spinal Injury Association Impairment Grade	Physical Findings
A: complete injury	no motor or sensory function below the level
B: incomplete injury	no motor function but sparing of some sensory function
C: incomplete injury	sparing of some motor function but with strength grade 3 or less for most muscles.
D: incomplete injury	sparing of some motor function but with strength grade 4 or 5 for most muscles.
E: minimal injury	normal motor and sensory findings

Table 3: American Spinal Injury Association Impairment Grades.

In cases of incomplete spinal cord damage, symptoms will vary based on the portion of the cord affected.

Central cord syndrome is the most common incomplete spinal cord injury syndrome. Central cord syndrome is most frequently seen after a fall in elderly patients who have a history of cervical spondylosis or spinal stenosis. Central cord syndrome results from a spinal cord contusion usually caused by hyperextension of the cervical spine. This contusion causes axonal disruption of the lateral columns selectively. Central cord syndrome affects fine motor control of the hands but may be seen distally as well, including loss of bladder control.

Anterior cord syndrome is characterized by complete motor paralysis and loss of temperature and pain perception distal to the lesion. Since posterior columns are spared, light touch, vibration, and proprioceptive input (sensation) are preserved. Anterior cord syndrome is caused either by direct compression or indirect injury to the anterior spinal artery. The region affected includes the descending corticospinal tract, ascending spinothalamic tract, and autonomic fibers. It is characterized by a corresponding loss of motor function, loss of pain and temperature sensation, and hypotension. This incomplete spinal cord syndrome has the worst prognosis, as only about 15% of patients regain motor function in recovery.

Brown-Séquard Syndrome is seen after damage to one side of the spinal cord, left or right, usually after penetrating trauma. It is associated with loss of function or impaired function on the side of the injury and altered pain and temperature loss on the opposite side of the injury. Among the incomplete spinal cord syndromes, Brown-Séquard has the best prognosis for functional recovery.

OBJECTIVE EVIDENCE

In any suspected spinal trauma, radiographic imaging is crucial. In most cases, CT scanning will be indicated for detailed assessment of the bony anatomy. MRI provides additional details about the spinal cord and surrounding soft tissues. In general, both studies are usually warranted. CT scans provide bony detail, and MRI provides information about the spinal cord and soft tissues.

A whole spine radiograph should be obtained to evaluate for any vertebral fractures. In the cervical spine, there are four parallel lines that should be assessed (see Figure 4). The anterior and posterior vertebral lines lie at the margin of the vertebral bodies front and back, respectively. The spinolaminar line defines the posterior margin of the spinal canal, and the posterior spinous line abuts the tips of the spinous processes. These lines should be smooth. Any so-called "step-off" is suspicious for ligamentous injury.

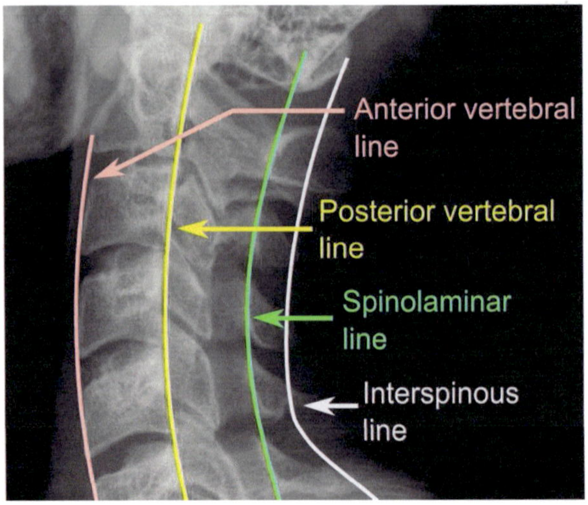

Figure 4: The "lines" of the cervical spine. (From https://upload.wikimedia.org/wikipedia/commons/1/10/X-ray_of_vertebral_lines.jpg)

For suspected instability of the cervical spine, patients who can move their heads on their own may have radiographs made in flexion/extension (see Figure 5) to assess stability.

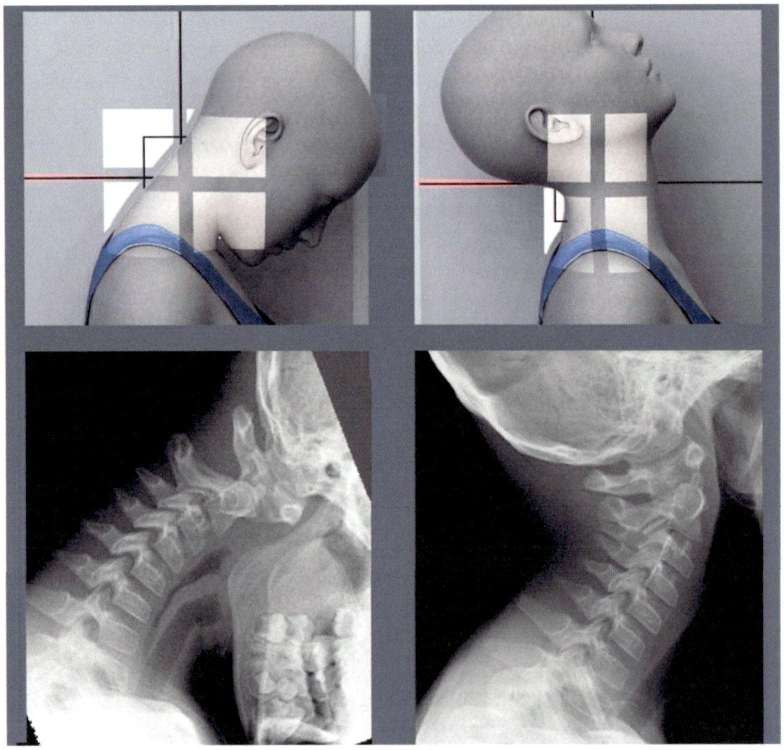

Figure 5: Flexion and extension radiographs of the cervical spine. Positioning and imaging are shown. These studies are normal: there is no step off in any of the four lines (see text) produced when the head is moved. (Modified from Radiopaedia.org, rID: 10338 and Radiopaedia.org, rID: 80305)

The open mouth view allows assessment of the odontoid process of C2 (see Figure 6).

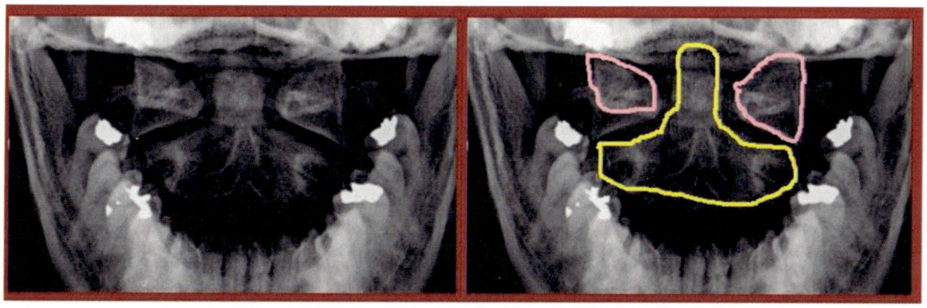

Figure 6: The open mouth view x-ray is to the left, in which normal anatomy is shown. In the annotated x-ray to the right, the lateral masses of C1 are in pink while C2 and its odontoid process are in yellow. (Case courtesy Radiopaedia.org, rID: 48418)

Although x-rays have been historically important, CT scans have replaced x-rays over the last two decades for the evaluation of bony injuries, given their higher resolution and sensitivity. CT scanning will detect most fractures (Figures 7 and 8). CT can also help evaluate the patency of the spinal canal, although direct visualization of the spinal cord is still poor.

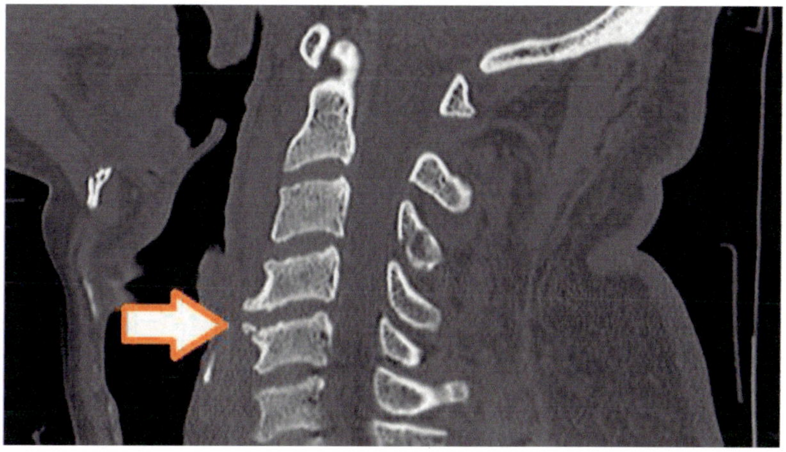

Figure 7: A CT scan showing a small fracture (arrow) through an anterior/superior osteophyte of C5. (Courtesy of Radiopedia)

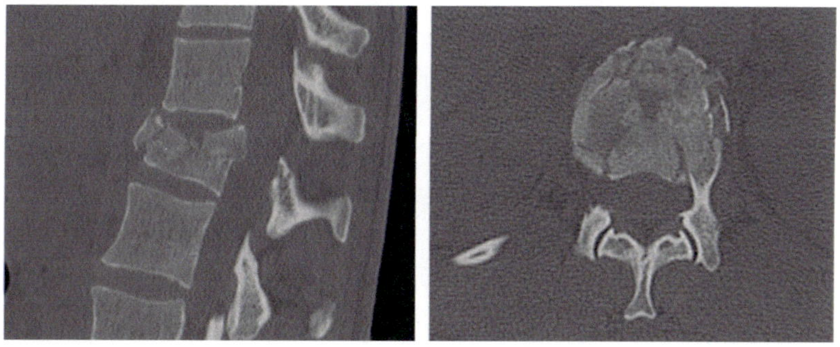

Figure 8: A CT scan of a thoracic fracture, seen in sagittal and axial CT images. The axial view to the right shows that the canal is patent. (Case courtesy of Radiopaedia.org, rID: 5274)

The main indications of MRI (see Figures 9 and 10) in spinal trauma include the following:

- X-ray or CT scan findings suggestive of ligamentous injury (e.g., spondylolisthesis or asymmetric disc space widening)
- Concern for epidural hematoma, disc herniation or occult fracture
- Suspected spinal cord abnormalities
- Suspected cervical instability in trauma patients who are obtunded or otherwise unable to pose for flexion/extension radiographs
- Neurological deficit detected on clinical examination.

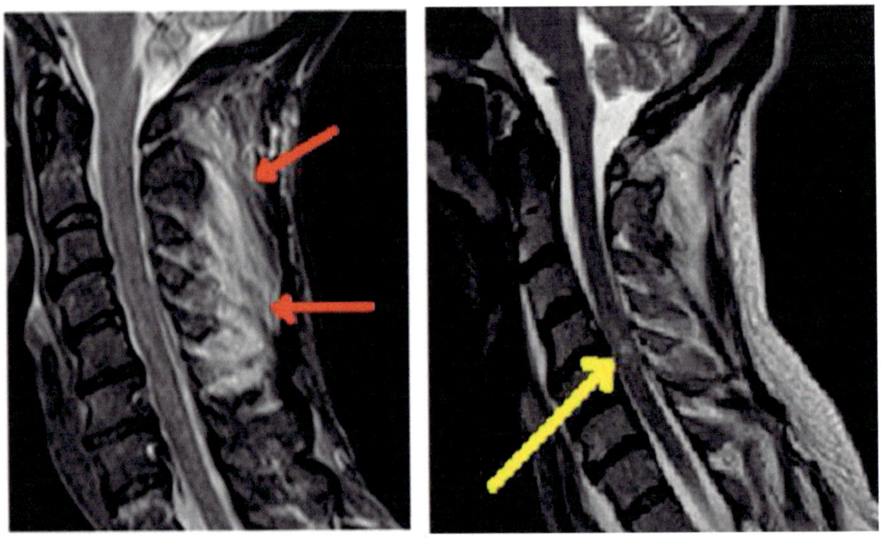

Figure 9: An MRI can be used to identify soft tissue abnormalities not apparent on radiography. On the left is an MRI showing interspinous ligament injury (red arrows). On the right, the yellow arrow points to a non-hemorrhagic contusion in the spinal cord. (Courtesy of BMC Musculoskelet Disordv.17; 2016PMC4957861)

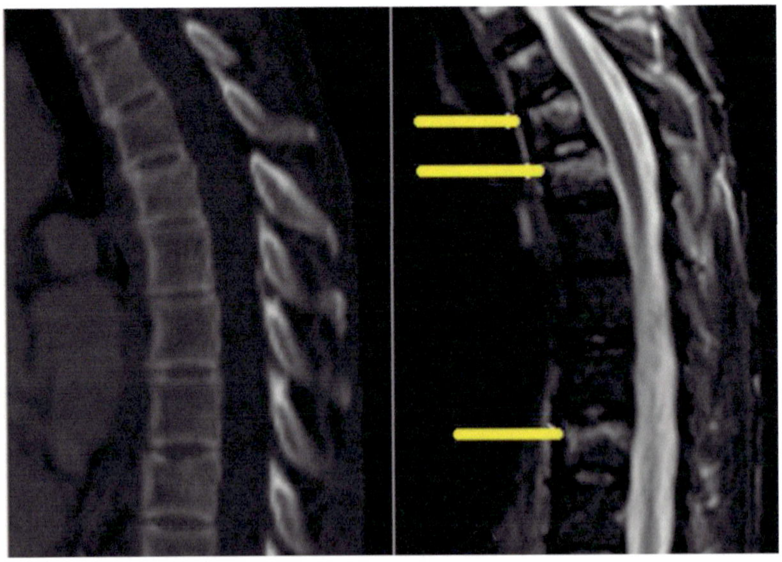

Figure 10: Sagittal CT image to the left did not show any sign of fracture but MRI (STIR) imaging of this patient shows bone marrow edema in the superior aspect of multiple vertebrae (yellow lines) suggesting bone contusions. (Courtesy of BMC Musculoskelet Disordv.17; 2016PMC4957861)

TREATMENT OPTIONS

Non-operative treatment of spinal trauma often centers on immobilization. Various immobilization devices can be used (see Figures 11 and 12), including a Philadelphia collar, a thoraco-lumbosacral orthosis, a lumbosacral corset, or a halo vest.

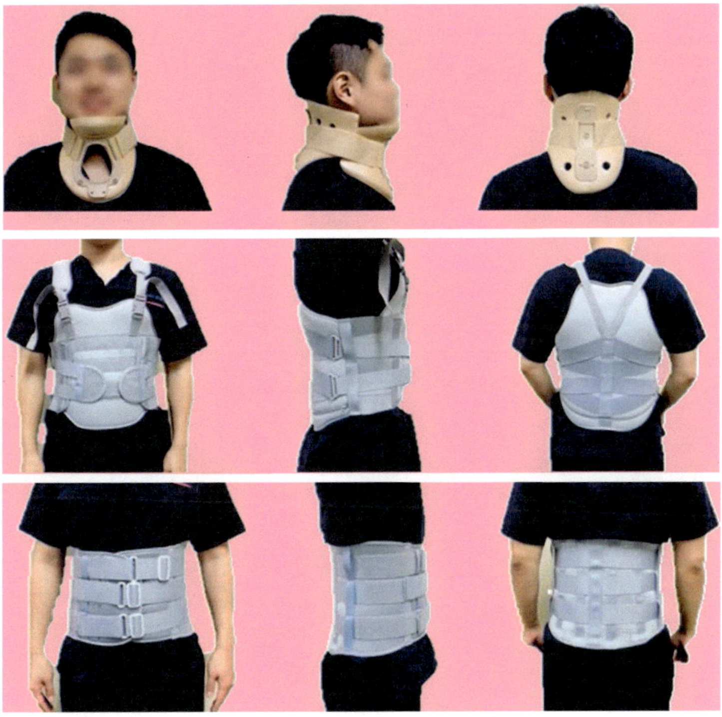

Figure 11: Philadelphia (cervical) collar, thoraco-lumbosacral orthosis, and lumbosacral corset. (Courtesy of Effectiveness of orthoses for treatment in patients with spinal pain doi: 10.12701/yujm.2020.00150 PMCID: PMC7142031)

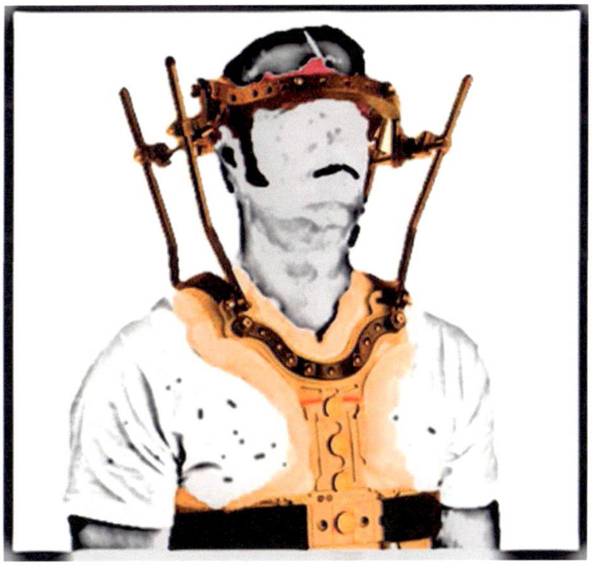

Figure 12: A halo vest is the most rigid form of external immobilization of the upper cervical spine. Fixation of the halo to a patient's head relies on pins spaced around a ring which are (after injection of a local anesthetic) tightened against the head above the orbits and ears.

Surgery for spinal trauma (see Figure 13), in general, consists of decompressing the spinal cord (that is, relieving any pressure on it) and stabilizing the spine, usually by a spinal fusion with plates, screws, wires or rods. The construct can be supplemented with bone graft.

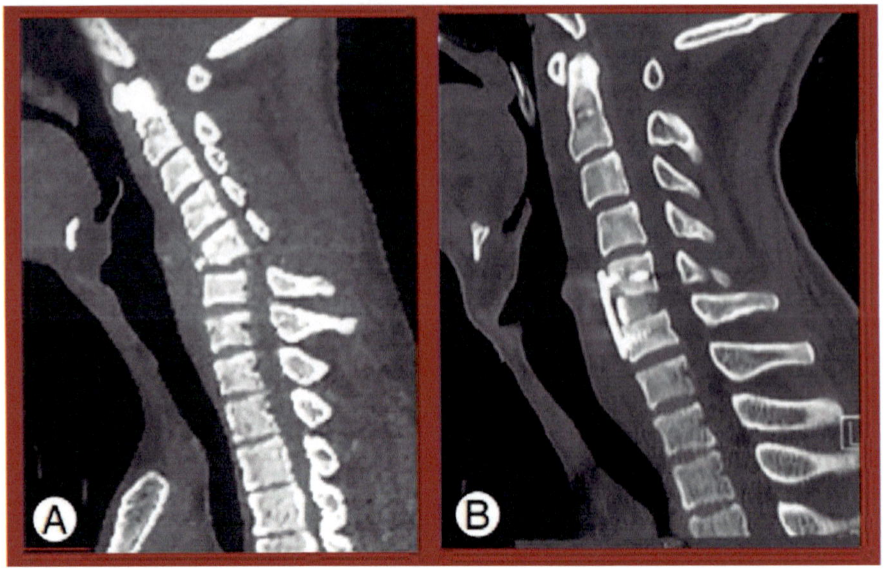

Figure 13: Preoperative CT midsagittal images of a right facet dislocation and left facet subluxation at the C5–C6 level. Images obtained after anterior cervical discectomy and fusion CT show an anterior plate holding the normal alignment of the facet joints. (From https://www.asianspinejournal.org/journal/view.php?number=1193)

Spinal trauma leading to spinal cord damage will require immediate administration of certain medications. These include prophylaxis for deep vein thrombosis and fluids or vasopressors to treat or prevent shock. Administration of steroids in an attempt to reduce spinal cord edema is controversial, especially in the setting of conditions such as poly-trauma or open fractures, where the risk infection is elevated. According to a meta-analysis in the journal *Neurology* published in 2019, high-dose methylprednisolone early after acute spinal cord injury "does not contribute to better neurologic recoveries but may increase the risk of adverse events."

CHAPTER 11.

SPINAL TRAUMA & SPINAL CORD INJURY: SPECIFIC INJURIES

In this section, a selection of notable spinal traumatic conditions will be reviewed: injuries to the upper cervical spine (C1, also known as the atlas and C2, the axis); lower (subaxial) cervical injuries; thoracolumbar fractures; and osteoporotic vertebral compression fractures. Injuries to the discs (including cauda equina syndrome) and spinal sprains and strains will be covered elsewhere.

ATLAS FRACTURES

Atlas fractures are rare. They are usually caused by compression to the top of the skull, with force transmitted on the atlas into the axis. If the force causes the lateral masses to split, the injury is known as a Jefferson fracture (Figure 1). Jefferson fractures are reduced by traction and immobilized for about 12 weeks. This mechanism of injury can also cause rupture of the transverse ligament which normally prevents the atlas from slipping forward relative to the axis. In cases where the transverse ligament is ruptured, surgical arthrodesis (fusion) of C1 to C2 is indicated. If there is a dislocation of C1/C2 due to transverse ligament rupture without fracture, projection of bone into the neural canal can cause immediate death and thus are not seen clinically.

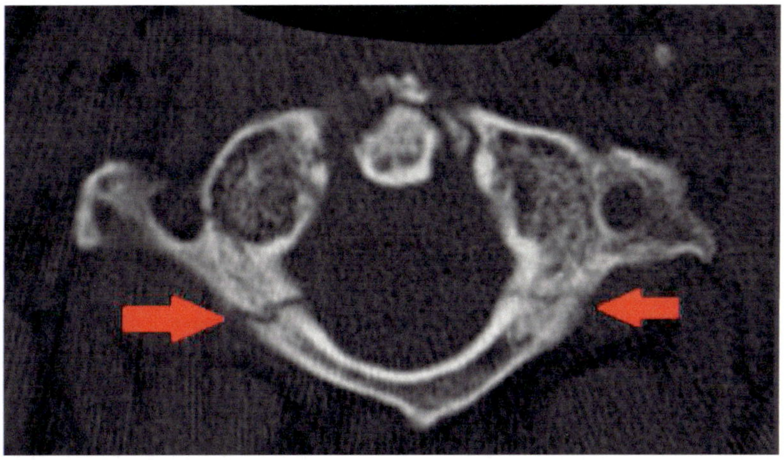

Figure 1: A Jefferson fracture. (From https://en.wikipedia.org/wiki/Jefferson_fracture)

ODONTOID FRACTURES

Odontoid fractures represent about 10% of cervical spine fractures and are the most common fracture of C2 itself. Odontoid fractures are seen in low energy falls in elderly patients. Odontoid fractures are also seen in younger patients after high energy mechanisms of injury causing cervical hyperflexion or hyperextension. Treatment is guided by the location of the fracture (Figure 2). Type I fractures are avulsions of the tip of the odontoid dens and are treated with a cervical orthosis. Type II fractures are at the junction of the odontoid and the body of C2. Younger patients can be treated with halo immobilization, but elderly people typically do not tolerate that and may need surgical stabilization. Surgery is more often chosen when there is comminution of the fracture or displacement or posterior angulation greater than about 5mm or 10 degrees, respectively. Surgery may also be especially indicated if there is a risk of poor bone healing (as suggested by a history of smoking or osteoporosis, for example). Type III fractures involve the body of the axis and are treated with immobilization because the cancellous bone typically heals.

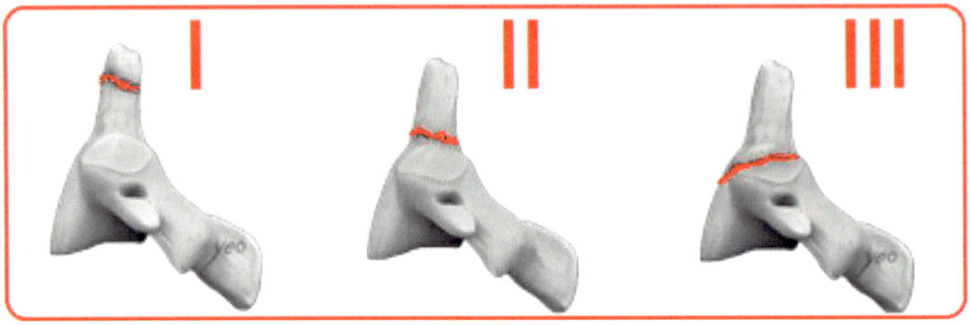

Figure 2: Odontoid fracture patterns. (Modified from Cho EJ, Kim SH, Kim WH, et al. Clinical Results of Odontoid Fractures according to a Modified, Treatment-Oriented Classification. Korean J Spine. 2017;14(2):44-49. doi:10.14245/kjs.2017.14.2.44 https://www.ncbi.nlm.nih.gov/pmc/articles/PMC5518434/)

An os odontoideum is a fragment that appears like a Type II odontoid fracture; it may represent failure of fusion during growth and development or may be a residual of prior trauma. It is managed by observation, without intervention. Os odontoideum is not uncommon in patients with Down Syndrome, and may be managed with observation or with surgery, depending upon the clinical situation.

HANGMAN'S FRACTURE

A hangman's fracture is a bilateral fracture of the C2 pars interarticularis with a traumatic spondylolisthesis (slippage) of C2 on C3 (Figure 3). It is the second most common fracture of the C2 vertebral body, excluding injuries to the dens. Although the name suggests a hyperextension and distraction mechanism of injury (as would be seen in a judicial execution), hyperextension with axial loading is the more common mechanism. Common mechanisms of injury include motor vehicle collisions, diving, or high-velocity contact sports. Despite the traumatic spondylolisthesis of C2/C3, a hangman's fracture rarely leads to spinal cord injury as the bony fractures, contrary to intuition perhaps, tend to increase the space for the spinal cord. A CT scan and MRI should be obtained to assess the fracture and soft tissues, respectively. Because the vertebral artery is at particular risk for injury with a hangman's fracture, angiography may also be needed. Nearly all cases of hangman's fracture can be managed successfully with immobilization with a halo or collar.

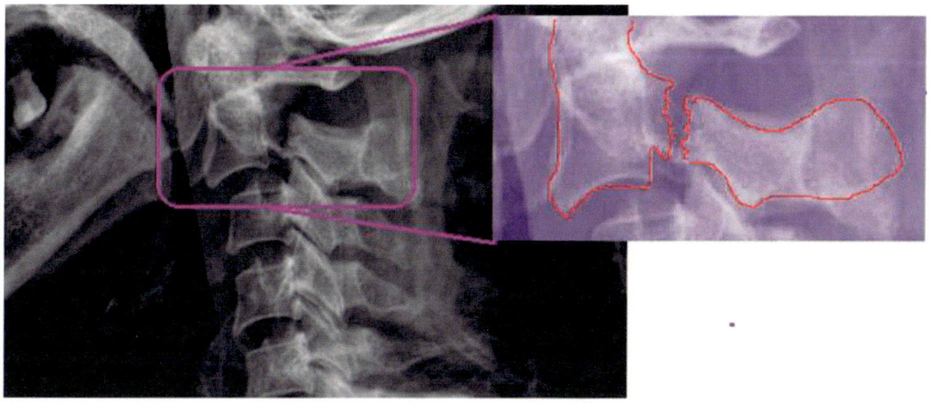

Figure 3: Hangman's fracture. (From https://josr-online.biomedcentral.com/articles/10.1186/s13018-020-01911-3)

EXTENSION TEARDROP FRACTURES

Extension teardrop fractures are small, stable avulsions that are usually not associated with cord injury (Figure 4). They are more commonly seen at C2. With forced extension of the neck, especially in the setting of stiffness caused by degenerative disease, there can be an avulsion of the anteroinferior aspect of the vertebral body with disruption of the anterior longitudinal ligament.

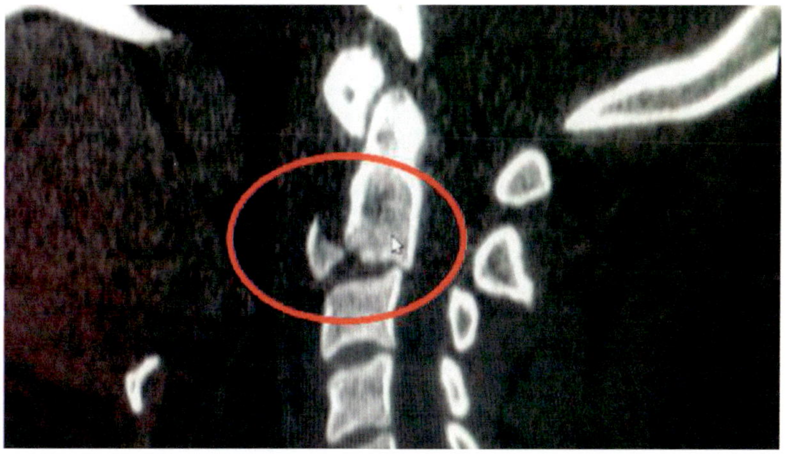

Figure 4: CT images of an extension teardrop fracture at C2. (Case courtesy of Dr M Venkatesh, Radiopaedia.org, rID: 26327)

It is important to not conflate extension teardrop avulsion fractures with the more serious flexion teardrop fractures seen in the lower cervical spine. Both manifest as a (teardrop-shaped) fragment fractured from the anteroinferior aspect of the vertebra. Critical differences are listed in the table below.

	Extension Teardrop Fracture	**Flexion Teardrop Fractures**
Common location	C2	C4-C7
Mechanism	Avulsion	Compression/Shearing
Ligament injury	Anterior longitudinal ligament	Posterior longitudinal ligament
Spinal Cord injury	Rare	More common
Stability	Stable in flexion	Unstable
Treatment	Non-operative	Surgical

Table 1: Extension Teardrop Fracture vs. Flexion Teardrop Fractures

CERVICAL FACET DISLOCATIONS

Cervical facet dislocations are often caused by a combination of flexion and distraction. They are seen in younger patients after high energy trauma such as motor vehicle accidents or contact sport collisions. Bilateral facet dislocation is characterized by 50% subluxation and is often associated with significant spinal cord injury. If rotational force is applied, it is possible to have only one facet dislocate (Figure 5). These unilateral dislocations are manifest with about 25% subluxation seen on x-ray and a single level nerve root injury. For example, a C6/7 unilateral dislocation presents with a C7 dysfunction: weakness, wrist flexion and numbness in the index and middle finger.

In addition to subluxation, there may be increased lordosis, soft tissue swelling, and widening of the interspinous distance. If subluxation is seen on plain films, the bony anatomy of the injury can be confirmed with a CT scan. An MRI is used to identify disk herniation, spinal cord compression or myelomalacia. An MRI can also detect spinal cord hematoma and any disruption of the supraspinous/interspinous ligaments and facet capsules.

If there is a bilateral facet dislocation with neurological deficits, and the patient is awake and cooperative, emergent closed reduction followed by urgent surgical stabilization is indicated. Closed reduction is carried out by gradually increased axial traction applied to tongs fixed to the skull with pins. If the patient is not awake and cooperative, MRI followed by open reduction is indicated. Stable, unilateral dislocations can be treated with immobilization alone.

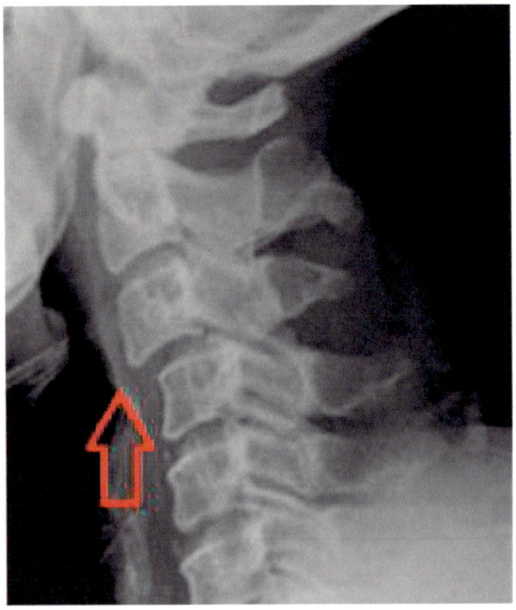

Figure 5: A C3-4 unilateral facet joint dislocation. Lateral radiographs of the cervical spine show unilateral facet joint dislocation with anterior displacement (red arrow). (From https://synapse.koreamed.org/articles/1037797)

CERVICAL BODY FRACTURES

Cervical body fractures (Figure 6) in the lower cervical vertebrae include "compression fractures," limited to the anterior vertebral body without retropulsion of bone into canal, or "burst fractures" which involve the posterior aspects of the body, with retropulsion of bone into the spinal canal and associated spinal cord injury. (The phrase "compression fractures" is surrounded by air quotes as it is referring to a specific pattern, as described. The mechanism of injury of other injuries may also involve "compression," in the general meaning of the word.)

Flexion teardrop fractures are caused by axial/flexion forces that compress the anterior-inferior aspect of the vertebra (usually C4, C5 or C6) and push the posterior portion of vertebra into the canal. They are associated with extensive injuries to both bone and ligament and thereby produce spinal instability. Associated spinal cord injury is common.

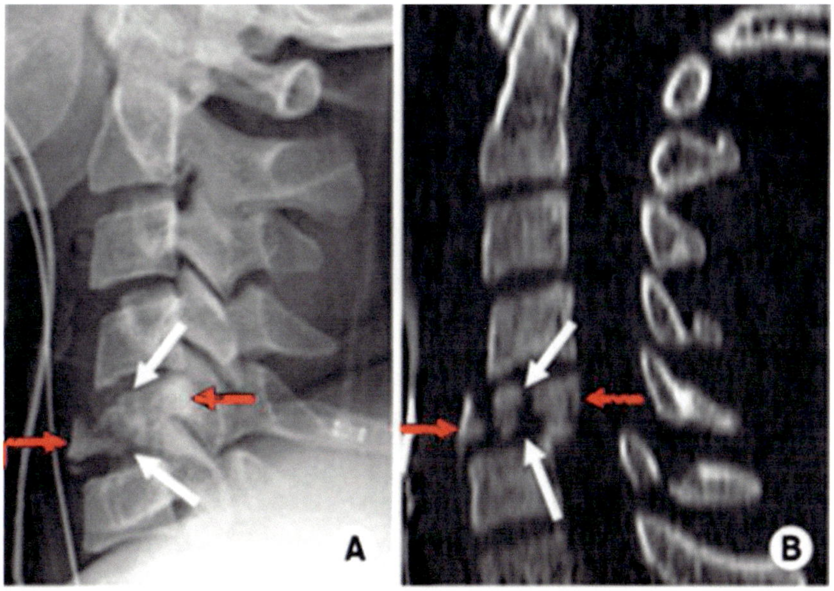

Figure 6: Cervical body fracture with anterior and posterior displacement. (From https://jkfs.or.kr/DOIx.php?id=10.12671/jkfs.2011.24.1.100)

THORACOLUMBAR FRACTURES

Thoracolumbar burst fractures (Figure 7) most commonly present with symptoms of spinal cord injury. Due to the location of the injury distal to the cervical nerve roots, only the lower extremities are affected. If the spinal canal is compromised by the retropulsion of the vertebral body, maximal compression of the spinal cord occurs at the moment of trauma. Neurologic symptoms can occur with burst fractures. In the rare cases without significant neurologic symptoms, the patient will complain of severe, focal back pain over the injured vertebrae. Mobility of the thoracolumbar junction is limited both by pain and instability.

Thoracolumbar burst fractures can be described in terms of their geographic limits: anterior, middle and posterior column injuries. Direct damage can be limited to the anterior column of the spine (anterior longitudinal ligament + anterior 2/3 of vertebral body) the anterior plus the middle column, which includes the posterior longitudinal ligament and posterior 1/3 of vertebral body; or the inclusion of the posterior column, containing the ligamentum flavum, the spinous processes, the pedicles and the posterior ligaments.

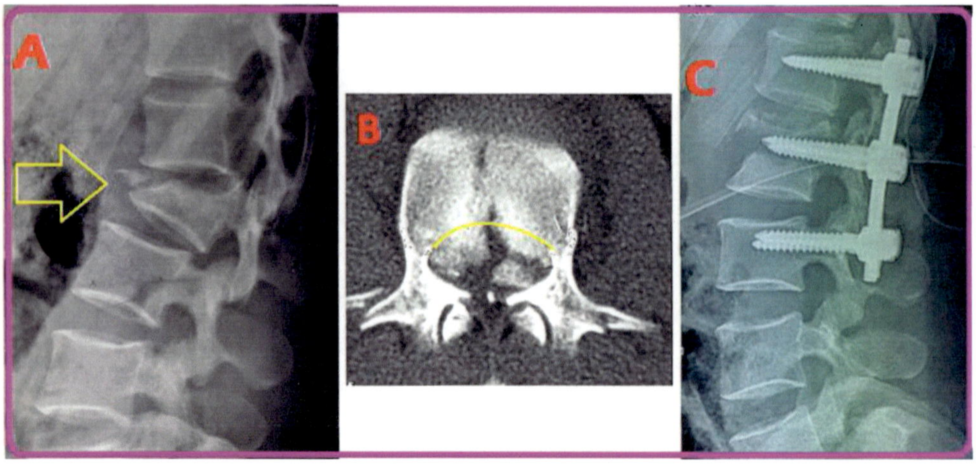

Figure 7: A) 35-year-old man with an L2 burst fracture; B) An axial computed tomography image shows comminution and canal encroachment; C) Two-level posterior fixation was done from L1 to L3. (From https://bmcmusculoskeletdisord.biomedcentral.com/articles/10.1186/s12891-020-3038-6 BMC Musculoskelet Disord 21, 17 (2020). https://doi.org/10.1186/s12891-020-3038-6)

OSTEOPOROSIS AND VERTEBRAL COMPRESSION FRACTURES

Osteoporosis is characterized by poor bone mineral density and a propensity for so-called "fragility fractures" of the distal radius, the hip, and the vertebral bodies. Of these three fragility fractures, vertebral compression fractures (Figure 8) are the most common, with an annual incidence of 700,000. It is estimated that one in four postmenopausal women will suffer a vertebral compression fracture in their lifetime. Vertebral compression fractures are responsible for more than $10 billion of health care expenditure annually in the USA and are a harbinger of increasing morbidity and mortality.

Most osteoporosis-related vertebral compression fractures are found in the thoracolumbar region (T12 to L2) in patients aged 50 to 60. (By contrast, wrist fractures are most common in the 5th decade and hip fractures are most common in the 7th decade.) In the case of a vertebral compression fracture, the onset pain is often insidious. If acute pain is noted, many patients may report that their pain started after a seemingly benign event like coughing, rolling over in bed, or lifting an object.

Physical exam for osteoporosis is unrevealing, but a secondary vertebral compression fracture can cause tenderness to palpation over the fracture level. Other signs of compression fracture include progressing loss of height, kyphotic deformity, or paraspinal muscle contraction (necessary to maintain posture).

It is unlikely that an osteoporosis-related vertebral compression fracture will cause any damage to the spinal cord. That is because the bone collapses on itself and does not create a mass effect in the central canal (as might be seen with a burst fracture of healthy bone in high energy trauma). The loss of height in the vertebral column may, however, compress the neural foramina and put pressure on exiting nerve roots.

Because vertebral compression fractures can also be caused by metastatic cancer or infection, it is important to exclude these diagnoses when the presentation is not typical for an osteoporosis-related fracture. Suspicion should be raised in patients with a known cancer history; patients under age 50, especially with no history of overt trauma; a history of weight loss, fevers, or other constitutional signs and symptoms (e.g., fever); a vertebral compression fracture located at the T5 vertebra or above; or risk factors for cancer or infection, such as smoking and immunosuppression, respectively.

A vertebral compression fracture is itself a red flag for the presence of osteoporosis, and a formal work-up (with treatment if the diagnosis is confirmed) should be initiated.

X-ray imaging of the entire spine should be performed in patients with suspected vertebral compression fractures. A 20% or 4mm loss of vertebral height is consistent with the diagnosis (see Figure 8). A CT scan may be obtained if radiography is inadequate or if there are lower extremity neurologic findings. Magnetic resonance imaging is needed only if there is a question about the chronicity of the fracture or the presence of a spinal cord injury.

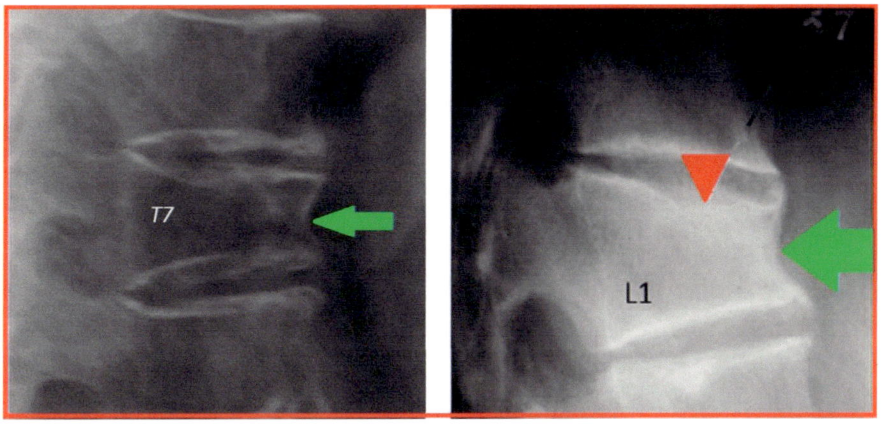

Figure 8: A vertebral compression fracture at L1 is shown at right. The red arrow points to an upper endplate fracture, and anterior cortex buckling is denoted by the green arrow. In the left panel, there is a T7 vertebral compression fracture with anterior cortex buckling also denoted by the green arrow, but there is no associated endplate fracture. (Images courtesy Osteoporotic vertebral endplate and cortex fractures: A pictorial review https://www.sciencedirect.com/science/article/pii/S2214031X18300986#fig3)

A history of at least one prior vertebral compression fracture increases risk of a future vertebral compression fractures by a factor of five. Risk of future vertebral compression fractures is 12 times greater in those with two or more previous vertebral compression fractures.

In patients with known osteoporosis of the spine, management of osteoporosis with light weight training, calcium and vitamin D supplementation, and bisphosphonate medications can reduce fracture risk by 25% to 75%.

Most patients with a vertebral compression fracture have a stable spine and thus can be treated non-operatively. Surgery is reserved for patients with continued severe back pain after six weeks of conservative therapy, although evidence of surgical intervention efficacy is limited. Operative management of a vertebral compression fracture is usually achieved with vertebroplasty or kyphoplasty (see Figure 9).

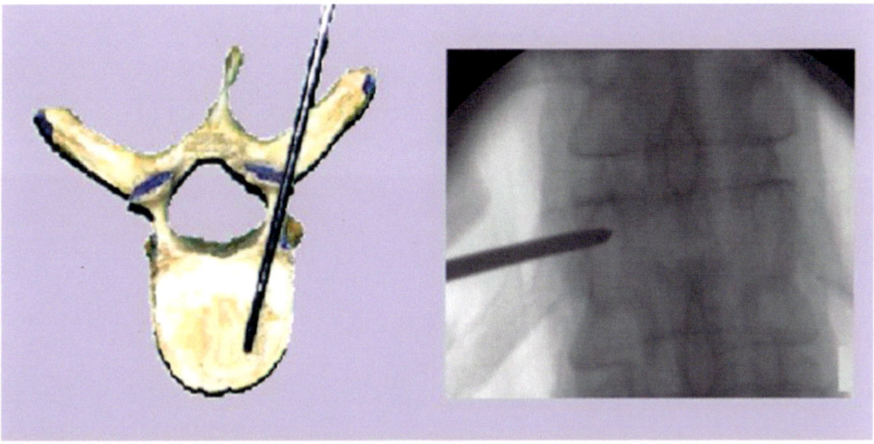

Figure 9: During kyphoplasty, a tube is introduced into the vertebral body (as shown in the cadaveric specimen in the left panel) under fluoroscopic guidance (right panel). A balloon is then passed through the tube and then inflated to restore the geometry of the fractured bone. The balloon is then removed, and the cavity is filled with polymethylmethacrylate to stabilizing the bone.

Rarely, surgical decompression and spinal stabilization with construct fixation are necessary to correct an injury to the posterior longitudinal ligament and prevent further deformity.

Vertebral compression fractures that produce kyphotic deformities can negatively impact pulmonary function by decreasing forced vital capacity when the kyphosis angle is greater than 70 degrees. This may also increase a patient's risk of developing atelectasis and pneumonia. Kyphosis can lead to GI symptoms such as constipation, early satiety, and even bowel obstruction due to the increase in abdominal cavity pressure. Vertebral compression fractures may cause poor balance (because the patient's center of gravity is tilted forward), leading to the potential for further falls. Loss of mobility leads to muscle atrophy and increases a patient's risk of DVT. Overall, vertebral compression fractures increase a patient's five-year mortality by 15%. One-year mortality for a vertebral compression fracture is 15% and 2-year mortality is 20%.

CHAPTER 12.

SPONDYLOLYSIS AND SPONDYLOLISTHESIS

Spondylolysis and spondylolisthesis are relatively common causes of low back pain, especially in young athletes. Spondylolysis refers to a weakening or other defect in a specific region of the vertebra called the pars interarticularis. These defects may be caused by repetitive stress. Spondylolisthesis refers to anterior slippage (displacement) of the vertebrae. This is often the result of bilateral spondylolysis, a so-called isthmic spondylolisthesis. Thus, spondylolysis and spondylolisthesis are separate yet interrelated conditions.

Besides isthmic spondylolisthesis, there are several other notable subtypes of spondylolisthesis. The two other most common forms are degenerative spondylolisthesis and dysplastic (congenital) spondylolisthesis. Less common forms include traumatic, pathologic, and iatrogenic/post-surgical.

STRUCTURE AND FUNCTION

The human spine has 24 vertebrae stacked one on top of the other: seven cervical, twelve thoracic and five lumbar. The lowest lumbar vertebra, L5, sits atop the sacrum. The vertebral bodies are separated by intervertebral discs, which function both as elastic bearings permitting motion as well as shock absorbers dissipating forces transmitted through the spinal column.

Behind the vertebral body lie the so-called posterior elements of the spine: the pedicles, the lamina and three processes: the transverse, the articular, and the spinous processes (Figure 1). The posterior elements connect to the vertebral body via the pedicles. At the dorsal limit of the pedicle is the pars interarticularis. The pars then extends cephalad to become the superior articular process and caudad to become the inferior articular process. The transverse process projects laterally from the pars in the thoracic and lumbar spine. Coursing dorsally from the pars, the laminae extend dorsally and medially to connect in the midline and complete the ring around the spinal canal. The spinous process is a dorsal extension from the junction of the two laminae at the midline.

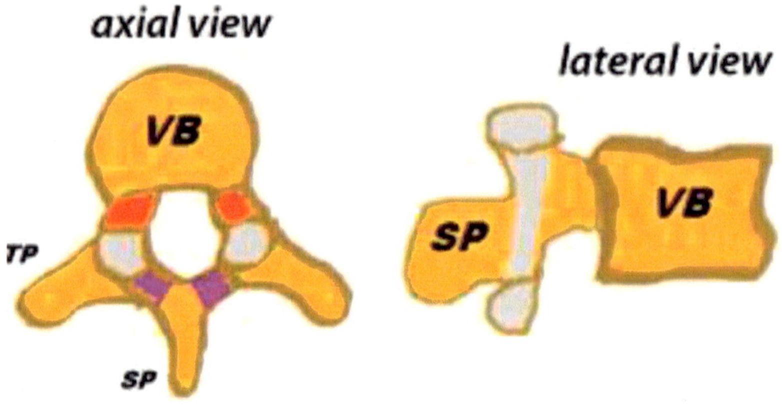

Figure 1: Schematic drawings of a lumbar vertebra, seen from above (axial view, on the left) and from the side (lateral view, right). VB: vertebral body; TP: transverse process (omitted from drawing on the right as it projects out of the plane); SP: spinous process. As seen from above, the central canal, behind the vertebral body, is surrounded by the pedicles (red), lamina (purple) and the superior and inferior articulating processes and the bone that connects them, the pars intraarticularis (gray).

Damage to the pars can incite an attempt at healing. The resultant hypertrophic fibrous tissue can cause foraminal stenosis with compression of the exiting nerve root. This most commonly occurs at L5-S1, resulting in an L5 radiculopathy.

On each side, left and right, the inferior articular processes of the vertebra above and the superior articular processes of the vertebra below, come together to form the facet joints. The function of the facet joint is to guide and also limit motion of the spine. Specifically, the facet joints in the lumbar spine permit flexion, extension, and rotation while simultaneously preventing extremes of these motions as well as translation.

Because the pars bridges the articular processes to the vertebral body, damage to the pars results in functional incompetence of the facet joints. It is this loss of restraint that allows anterior displacement or "slippage" of the superior vertebral body: spondylolisthesis (Figure 2).

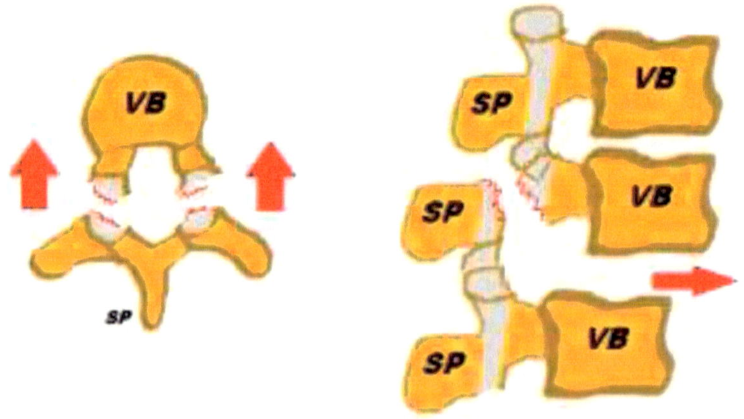

Figure 2: If there is a pars defect, the bodies above can slip forward relative to the body below.

In the vast majority of cases, spondylolysis is a developmental defect that may be present in up to 5-7 percent of the population and is typically asymptomatic. In the setting of new onset low back pain, spondylolysis may occur from overuse causing microfracture. In rare circumstances, a fracture in the pars articularis can occur following an acute load or trauma.

While the progression from a pars defect to spondylolisthesis is the mechanism of isthmic type spondylolisthesis, the pathophysiology of degenerative spondylolisthesis is different. In the most fundamental sense, the major difference between isthmic and degenerative forms is the *absence* of a defect in the pars interarticularis causing the anterior displacement in degenerative spondylolisthesis. Instead, the pathophysiology in degenerative spondylolisthesis centers around degeneration of the facet joint and intervertebral discs, leading to instability and increased motion of the vertebra. Degenerative spondylolisthesis is most commonly seen at L4-L5. Because the pars remains intact, the posterior elements of the sliding vertebra must also slide as a unit. Thus, degenerative spondylolisthesis is more likely to result in stenosis within the canal (especially the subarticular region) affecting the traversing roots. This contrasts with the isolated foraminal stenosis typically encountered with isthmic spondylolisthesis.

With respect to the other, rarer forms of spondylolisthesis, the dysplastic (congenital) type occurs secondary to abnormal spine development in utero, traumatic is the result of severe traumatic injury leading to vertebral displacement, and pathologic refers to the presence of a secondary disease process resulting in instability and displacement of the vertebra, including osteoporosis, malignancy, or infection.

PATIENT PRESENTATION

The diagnosis of spondylolysis is often an incidental discovery on an x-ray without any clinical signs or symptoms. In fact, the majority of patients with radiographic evidence of spondylolysis are asymptomatic.

In patients with spondylolysis that have symptoms, however, the most common complaint is low back pain of gradual onset that is worsened with activity, especially activities which involve hyperextension of the lumbar spine. The quality of the pain is non-specific and may resemble that of an ordinary lumbar muscle strain.

The presentation of isthmic spondylolisthesis is similar to that of spondylolysis, with non-specific low back pain often being the primary complaint. In spondylolisthesis, however, there is a higher occurrence of radicular symptoms. Impingement of the L5 nerve root in the foramen is most common, resulting in radiculopathy (paresthesias or pain radiating to the legs, or "sciatica").

In rare circumstances, patients with spondylolisthesis can experience a "*listhetic* crisis" characterized by severe back pain, neurologic deficits, and hamstring spasm, all which may be exacerbated by extension of the lumbar spine.

On physical examination of patients with spondylolysis and spondylolisthesis, there may be evidence of increased lumbar lordosis (inward curvature of the spine), decreased range of motion of the spine, pain upon lumbar spine extension, or a palpable step off of the spinous process (representing anterior displacement in spondylolisthesis). They may also have sensory or motor findings on neurologic exam depending upon any underlying neural compression.

In degenerative spondylolisthesis, low back pain is the most common symptom as well. These patients, however, may experience neurogenic claudication and leg pain secondary to spinal canal stenosis, which is more common in the degenerative than the isthmic form.

OBJECTIVE EVIDENCE

The gold standard modality for the diagnosis of spondylolysis and spondylolisthesis are plain radiographs of the lumbar spine. The important views are standing anterior-posterior (AP) and lateral in the standing position. Oblique views may also be obtained, but these are unnecessary in most cases.

In the AP view, sclerosis of the pars interarticularis may be appreciated secondary to stress reaction. From the lateral view, a defect in the pars interarticularis is identifiable in the majority of cases (Figure 3).

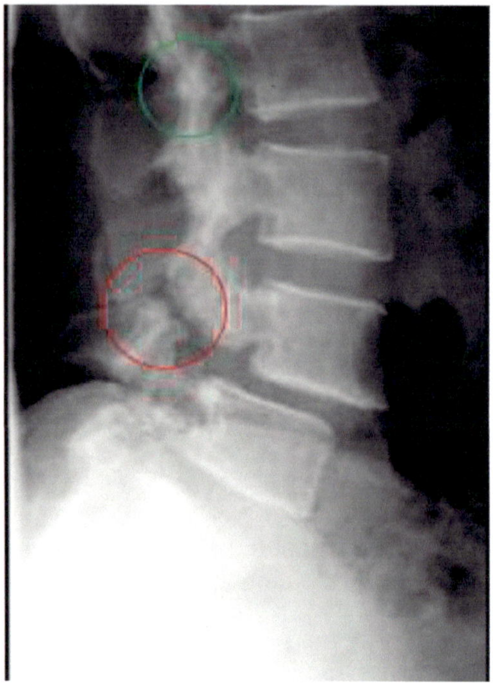

Figure 3: A pars defect is shown in the red circle; a normal pars is seen above in the green circle. (Case courtesy of Radswiki, Radiopaedia.org, rID: 11967)

The oblique film is a more specific view in the assessment of spondylolysis and spondylolisthesis. From this angle, the vertebra in the lumbar spine demonstrate the classic "Scottie dog" appearance (Figure 4), consisting of the superior articular process (ears of the dog), transverse process (head), isthmus (neck), lamina and spinous process (body), and inferior articular processes (foreleg and hindleg). In spondylolysis, the defect in the pars interarticularis appears as a neck collar on the Scottie dog.

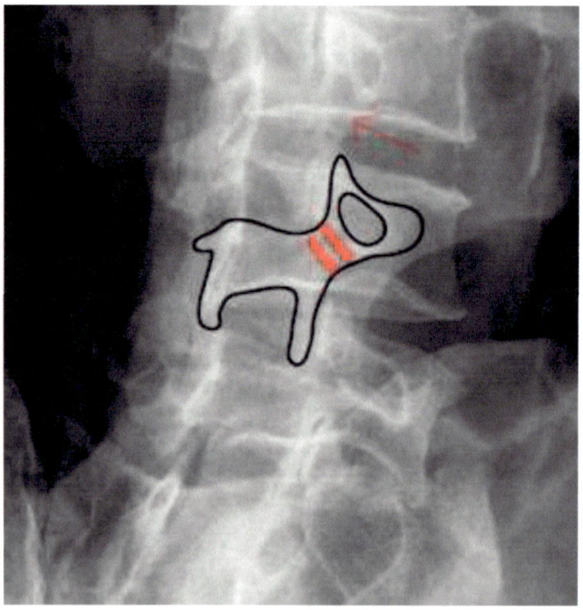

Figure 4: An oblique view of the lumbar spine, showing the "Scottie Dog." The pars is represented by the dog's collar, shown in faint red here. (Case courtesy of A.Prof Frank Gaillard, Radiopaedia.org, rID: 7552)

In spondylolisthesis, there is relative anterior displacement of the superior articular process, allowing the entire body to slip forward (Figure 5).

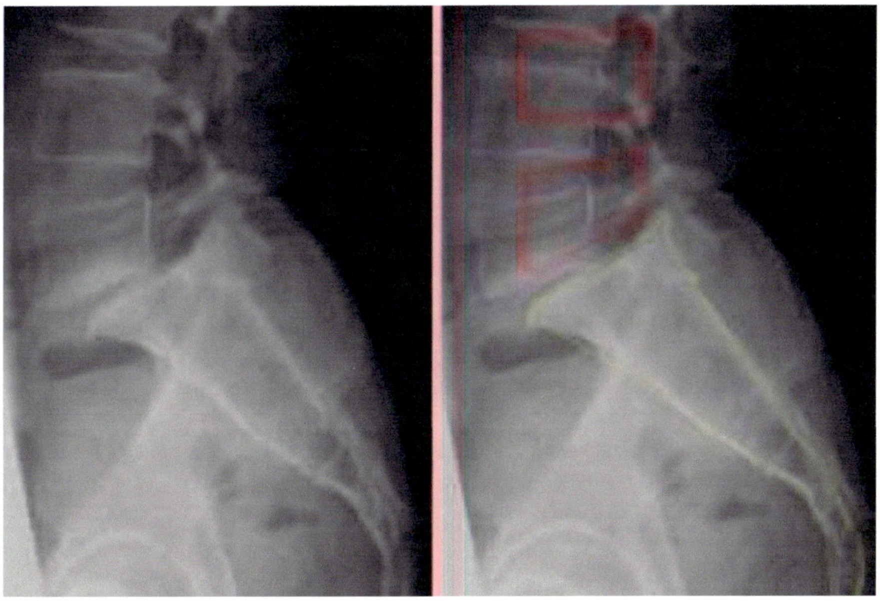

Figure 5: At left is a lateral x-ray showing an anterolisthesis at the L5-S1 level. In the annotation at right, the sacrum is outlined in yellow and the lumbar vertebral bodies in purple. The faint red lines outline the correct anatomic position from which the lumbar bodies have slipped. (Modified from https://en.wikipedia.org/wiki/Spondylolisthesis#/media/File:SpondylolisthesisL5S1.jpg)

Spondylolisthesis can be graded based on magnitude of vertebral displacement. The superior endplate of the caudal vertebra is divided into quarters. The grade is dependent on location of the poster-inferior corner of the vertebra above. Grade 1 represents a 0-25% displacement, grade 2: 25-50%, grade 3: 50-75%, and grade 4: > 75%. Grades 1 and 2 are considered 'low grade' and grades 3 and 4 are considered 'high grade'. This distinction is important when developing an appropriate treatment strategy.

Advanced imaging may also play a role in the assessment of spondylolysis and spondylolisthesis in select circumstances. CT scan is the best modality for revealing the specific anatomy of the underlying lesion in spondylolysis, and thus can be helpful for delineating subtle defects. In patients with neurologic complaints or deficits on examination, MRI is warranted to further assess for neural element impingement. Bone scan (SPECT) is also highly sensitive for spondylolysis, and may be utilized in patients with a high suspicion for a pars defect with normal or inconclusive radiographs in whom cross-sectional imaging is undesirable.

EPIDEMIOLOGY

While the precise etiology of spondylolysis remains unknown, the pars defects typically occur in childhood or adolescence as an acquired phenomenon, as true congenital spondylolysis is exceedingly rare. This anatomic variant is present in 5 to 7 percent of the entire population, but can occur in as many as 45 percent of pediatric athletes involved in high risk sports. (High risk activities include gymnastics, Olympic weightlifting, football, dancing, figure skating, and wrestling.) This is currently the most common identifiable source of low back pain in adolescents.

Progression of spondylolysis to spondylolisthesis is uncommon, occurring in less than 15 percent of patients. Certain anatomic risk factors can help predict which patients are at increased risk of progressive listhesis.

L5-S1 is the most commonly affected spinal segment in isthmic spondylolisthesis (90%), followed by L4-L5 (10%).

Degenerative spondylolisthesis occurs in older adults. In the majority of cases, this occurs after the age of 40, though risk increases upon increasing age.

Isthmic spondylolisthesis is slightly more common in males, while degenerative spondylolisthesis is significantly more common in females (about eight times more prevalent) and occurs in approximately 10% of all women.

DIFFERENTIAL DIAGNOSIS

In the patient with unknown spondylolysis or spondylolisthesis presenting with low back pain, the differential diagnosis is broad. In the pediatric patient, this includes lumbar disc related pathology, lumbar muscle strain, Scheuermann's kyphosis, scoliosis, sacroiliac joint dysfunction, tumors (including especially osteoid osteoma), or infection (vertebral osteomyelitis or discitis). In the older patient, the differential diagnosis is similar but also includes degenerative disc disease or spinal stenosis without spondylolisthesis.

In a patient with confirmed spondylolisthesis, the differential diagnosis revolves around the specific etiology, and includes the six different types: dysplastic, isthmic, degenerative, traumatic, pathologic, and iatrogenic.

RED FLAGS

Pain that fails to relieve predictably with rest ("night pain") and associated constitutional symptoms (fever, chills, unintended weight loss) are always red flags for further investigation to avoid delays in making important diagnoses, such as malignancy or infection.

Signs or symptoms of cauda equina syndrome, which is a surgical emergency, include bowel or bladder incontinence, saddle anesthesia, and progressive lower extremity weakness. (Note that cauda equina compression from a high-grade listhesis requires translation of the posterior elements and laminae along with the body. Accordingly, compressions is highly unlikely in the setting of true isthmic spondylolisthesis.

TREATMENT OPTIONS AND OUTCOMES

The primary goal of treatment of spondylolysis is resolution of symptoms and return to activity. Radiographic healing of the pars defect may or may not correlate with the resolution of symptoms and is of secondary importance in the setting of isolated spondylolysis or low-grade spondylolisthesis.

There are three general categories of management strategy for patients with spondylolysis and spondylolisthesis: symptomatic treatment with analgesics and observation without activity modification/limitation (benign neglect); activity modification/limitation with or without bracing; and surgical intervention.

Benign neglect is most appropriate for asymptomatic or minimally symptomatic patients with isolated spondylolysis or low-grade spondylolistheses.

Activity modification is generally indicated for patients with spondylolysis or low-grade spondylolisthesis who are symptomatic. This strategy encompasses use of NSAIDs for pain control and physical therapy with a focus on stretching, lumbar spine flexion, core strengthening/stability as first-line.

For radicular pain that fails to improve with time and NSAID use, steroid injections may be a useful alternative.

Lumbar spine bracing may also be beneficial, particularly in the case of a failed trial of physical therapy or in an acute pars stress reaction spondylolysis, for which bracing is superior to activity restriction alone.

Surgical management is the final line of therapy for spondylolysis and spondylolisthesis. Surgery is rarely required for isolated spondylolysis without spondylolisthesis. Broadly, the major indications for surgery include refractory radicular symptoms, a progressive neurologic deficit, high grade progressive spondylolisthesis, and intractable pain or disability despite exhaustive non-operative management.

The goal of surgery for spondylolisthesis is to stabilize the unstable segment. This can prevent slip progression and reduce back or leg pain. Direct repair of a pars fracture may be considered in the absence of listhesis and at levels L4 and above in an effort to preserve lumbar motion. In degenerative spondylolisthesis, surgical options also typically include decompression (to address neural impingement) with or without concurrent fusion.

In general, the prognosis of spondylolysis and spondylolisthesis is very favorable. For symptomatic patients who undergo non-operative or operative treatment, the vast majority experience total relief of their pain and regain full functionality.

For patients with symptomatic spondylolysis, the majority will improve with observation and non-operative management. Only 15% of patients with spondylolysis will go on to develop spondylolisthesis.

For spondylolisthesis, the outcome is dependent upon grade/severity and specific subtype. Since most cases of spondylolisthesis are low grade, the overall prognosis is good. In these mild cases, non-operative management is successful in about 80% of patients. With regard to risk for displacement progression, dysplastic portends the highest rate (over 30%), while the most common type (isthmic) progresses in less than 5% of cases.

Severe spondylolisthesis portends a slightly worse prognosis, but the prognosis is still favorable overall. There is a higher risk of neurologic damage secondary to nerve compression, in addition to the risks associated with surgery (below). There is also a higher likelihood of persistent low back pain and disability, though surgery is successful in 85-90% of cases.

Specific complications of surgery include mainly pseudoarthrosis, infection, dural tear, neurologic deficits, and instrumentation (ie, the surgical hardware) failure. The risk of complications is generally higher for patients with degenerative spondylolisthesis given their increased age and medical comorbidities.

Note that excessive avoidance of activity may also impose costs on patients including deconditioning, weight gain, osteoporosis, and psychologic distress. It may be possible, thus, to be excessively conservative in recommending treatment.

RISK FACTORS AND PREVENTION

The primary risk factor for spondylolysis and spondylolisthesis is frequent hyperextension of the lumbar spine. Participation in sports such as gymnastics and football (and others in which the spine is extended) is associated with a higher prevalence of defects in the pars interarticularis.

The best approach for preventing spondylolysis is to avoid repetitive hyperextension of the lumbar spine. In addition, maintaining core muscle strength, flexibility and good bone health are important.

KEY TERMS

Spondylolysis, spondylolisthesis, facet joint, pars articularis, 'Scottie dog', spinal fusion

SKILLS

Understand the similarities and differences in the pathophysiology underlying spondylolysis and spondylolisthesis. Recognize the different subtypes and severity grading system for spondylolisthesis. Understand the non-operative and operative treatment modalities and their efficacy in the treatment of spondylolysis and spondylolisthesis.

Made in the USA
Monee, IL
05 November 2026

67384984R00064